# DESIGNING THE WORLD'S BEST:
# Children's Hospitals

# DESIGNING THE WORLD'S BEST:
# Children's Hospitals

images
Publishing

**Bruce King Komiske,** FACHE, Editor

in cooperation with **The National Association of Children's Hospitals and Related Institutions, HKS, Karlsberger Companies, NBBJ, & Shepley Bulfinch Richardson and Abbott**

First published in Australia in 1999 by
The Images Publishing Group Pty Ltd
ACN 059 734 431
6 Bastow Place, Mulgrave, Victoria 3170, Australia
Telephone: +(61 3) 9561 5544 Facsimile: +(61 3) 9561 4860
E-mail: books@images.com.au

National Library of Australia Cataloguing-in-Publication Data


Designing the World's Best: Children's Hospitals


ISBN 1 86470 042 4


1. Children - Hospitals. 2. Children - Hospitals - Pictorial works.
3. Hospital architecture. 4. Hospital architecture - Pictorial
works. 5. Hospitals - Design and construction. 6. Hospitals -
Design and construction - Pictorial works. I. Komiske, Bruce K.


725.57


Designed by The Graphic Image Studio Pty Ltd
Mulgrave, Australia


Film separations by Scanagraphix Pty Ltd


Printed in Hong Kong

# Contents

# The Purpose

The purpose of this book is two-fold. First, it is intended to serve as a unique reference guide for teams of healthcare and design professionals, as well as parents who engage in the exciting journey of creating a 'healing environment' as they plan the construction or renovation of a children's hospital or pediatric unit. The images and stories shared by others who have recently gone through this challenging process are meant to create a vision of what 'can be' if leadership teams encourage involvement and make a commitment to exceed expectations.

The second purpose of this book is to recognize the outstanding efforts of teams throughout the world for their contributions to healthcare and design. As a result of their creativity and multiple skills, millions of children and their families have the advantage of receiving care in an environment that enhances the healing process for many years to come.

**Bruce King Komiske, FACHE**
Executive Director
Children's Hospital Foundation
Westchester Medical Center, Valhalla NY

# The Challenge

As the president and CEO of the National Association of Children's Hospitals and Related Institutions, I have had the privilege of visiting over 120 children's hospitals in the United States, Canada and several other countries throughout the world. Unlike adult hospitals, planners and architects of children's hospitals are challenged to accommodate adults while at the same time, appeal to children of all ages—stimulating them intellectually, but calming them emotionally to assist the healing process.

The very best children's hospital environments instantly make a child feel at home, but with the license afforded by children's imagination, provide a touch of whimsy and surprise, delighting the child (and each of us), during a most critical time in their lives. Good design brings imagination and creativity to the forefront and does make a significant difference in the healing process.

The involvement of children and their families in the design process provides a creative spark, along with the functionality that doctors, nurses, and other health professions contribute by their participation. One hope for this book is that by presenting a catalog of exciting ideas and visions of some of the best designed children's hospitals in the world, future teams of professionals will be even more creative and successful in their endeavors. Let your imagination wander as you view these photos and help bring together not only the bricks and mortar but the spirit and soul of an organization to heal physically, mentally, and spiritually.

**Lawrence A. McAndrews, FACHE**
President & CEO
National Association of Children's Hospitals
and Related Institutions, Alexandria VA

# The Ten Guiding Principles of a Successful Project

1. **Vision** - No institution can afford to spend critical capital on a new facility and end up with the same program in a new box. Consider starting any new project with a one- or two-day retreat to which all potential stakeholders are invited and the emphasis is on brainstorming the 'ideal' and creating a vision that will exceed expectations. Clearly identify the value and strategic advantage you are striving to achieve as a result of the project. Break paradigms.

2. **Team approach** - The more individuals who have been involved in a project and will consider it their own, the more you have guaranteed the project's success. Identify all who have a stake in the outcome and organize them into multiple teams. Leadership of each team is critical, as is the need to clearly communicate between all involved. The individual with ultimate responsibility for the project should be a facilitator as opposed to a manager.

3. **Empowerment** - Once the teams are designated, they must be empowered to succeed. As the overall facilitator, it may be scary not to know every detail and it requires a great deal of trust. However, the ultimate project will be successful by reflecting the best of many motivated individuals. Some critical tools to ensure success of empowerment include: team minutes, 'back-planning schedules' that are strictly tracked, monthly cost summary reports with early warnings, creation of an operations document and detailed move task lists.

4. **Creativity** - This element is essential in the creation of a successful children's hospital. There is no additional cost for it and there is a significant loss without it. The importance of creativity must be conveyed from the project leadership and embraced by all involved, including the design team. Visits to exemplary children's hospitals will help in understanding both the need and value of this element.

**5.** **Involvement** - There are few events in the life of a community or region that can generate involvement and excitement more than the creation of a new children's hospital. Take full advantage of this involvement to significantly enhance the future success of the project. Reaching out to schools, clubs, the corporate world, the art community, local celebrities, and any other community organization results not only in capital dollars and ongoing operating support, but vests them in the continued success of the hospital for the future.

**6.** **Evaluation / Feedback** - Constantly provide opportunities for feedback, whether it be in the form of evaluations of team meetings as a standing agenda item, written evaluations of any larger meetings or brainstorming sessions. Offer opportunities for all constituencies to provide constructive feedback during each phase of the design process. This is most important for the hospital board, staff, and the Family Advisory Council. Consider creating a report card with detailed criteria that the leadership will use to evaluate the project at its conclusion and track your progress against these criteria. Also incorporate a post-occupancy evaluation process approximately a year after opening to measure your success and further improve the completed project.

**7.** **Exceed Expectations** - Ninety-nine percent of project resources and effort go to creating the expected result—a state-of-the-art, efficient, attractive facility that provides excellent service. The goal of a truly successful project, however, is to not only achieve these results but to constantly look for opportunities to go beyond the expected and delight and exceed expectations. In most instances, these elements of a project cost nothing other than looking for and creating these opportunities. These are the unexpected features that children and parents will talk about long after they have left the hospital.

**8.** **Communicate-Communicate-Communicate** - You cannot over communicate when it comes to project management. Use every resource from walking rounds throughout the hospital on all shifts, to a monthly project newsletter, or major display area in the hospital where the most current information will always be available. Despite the best of efforts, assume the majority of your constituencies still don't know the latest information and provide new opportunities for sharing it.

**9.** **'Parents as Partners'** - Participation of a parent in the creation of a new children's hospital occurs because either they are asked or they are angry. Make sure your organization is proactive in getting a group of parents involved in the planning early on in the process. The Child Life Department or Pediatric Nursing is an excellent source for parents of children that are chronically ill and use the hospital frequently. Over time, this group will hopefully become more organized, particularly if they feel that their input is valued and incorporated into the process. It is also essential that the design team is sensitive to receiving their input and values feedback from these most important stakeholders. Also, note that the involvement of the parents is in an advisory capacity only, with the hospital leadership and the board having ultimate responsibility.

**10.** **Celebrate** - Anyone involved in the healthcare industry today knows that it is a challenging time where the emphasis seems to be constantly on doing more with less. At times, there seems to be little to celebrate on a day-to-day basis. Take full advantage of the excitement, energy and hope for the future that a major new project brings to a medical center. Use all opportunities such as the team retreats, ground-breaking, topping off party, pre-opening open-houses, the move, and each birthday after opening to celebrate and give thanks for all involved. This approach will pay major dividends for many years to come.

**Bruce King Komiske, FACHE**
Executive Director
Children's Hospital Foundation
Westchester Medical Center, Valhalla NY

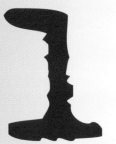

# Exterior Design

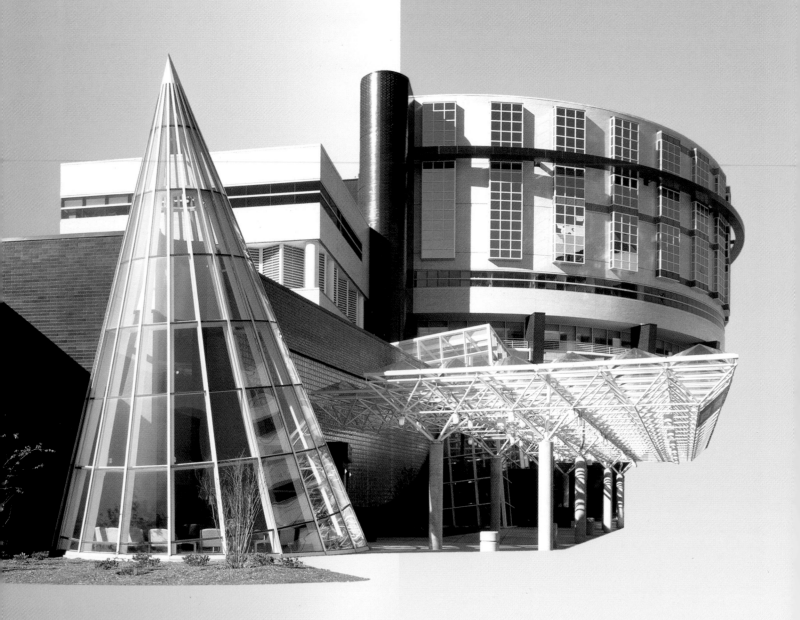

Children represent a unique end-user, especially in the design of an environment that supports healing. Designers need to create children's healthcare facilities that allow a supportive, healing, playful atmosphere for children while remaining technically and functionally precise. This philosophy must also incorporate the needs of families, staff, and community.

Today's children's healthcare facilities are focusing on transporting kids and their families into a world of healing, caring, and education. To promote this environment, a building's exterior design should evoke an inviting, non-threatening image. A playful, positive atmosphere should incorporate various elements of scale, color, texture, landscaping and light. There are also unique challenges when designing children's hospitals in urban versus suburban settings. Streetscape level elements provide the design focal point for urban children's hospitals while suburban facilities can establish an individual palette of design elements created to meet specific goals and objectives.

The exterior design of children's healthcare facilities is ideally articulated into smaller parts of solid and void, color and texture and shadow and light. Changes in material, color, and texture can create visual interest as well as help identify various care delivery areas. It is important to use colors that are suitable to the environment, climate, and location. Trendy, pop colors

can diminish in interest and intensity over a period of time. The use of touchable, textured exterior materials can help create an approachable building. Varying textures, including rough-cut stone, brick, steel, and glass can attract interest and create depth. The feeling of safety must also be of utmost importance in the design process. A safe image can be projected during the day and night by illuminating the entire facility from the entry to the parking lots. The use of varied lighting helps to create safe and playful areas. Landscaping adds visual interest, color and natural settings for children's hospitals. The use of trees, flowers, shrubs, topiary animals, water elements, and shaded seating areas help create a healing environment. Once inside, the interior elements should complement the exterior through the use of similar design vocabulary, colors, and textures.

Today's hospital planners are demonstrating the ability to plan and design with the child and family at the forefront. Only with forward-thinking will healthcare providers, consultants, and designers of children's healthcare facilities continue to promote safety, health and family support from the building's exterior to its interior.

Joseph G. Sprague, FAIA
HKS, Dallas TX

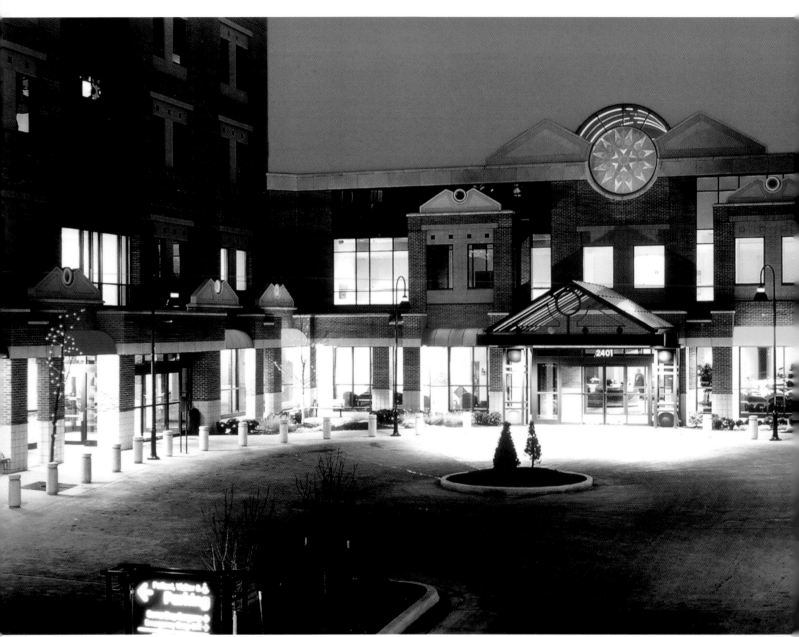

Children's Mercy Hospital, Kansas City MO
© Children's Mercy Hospital

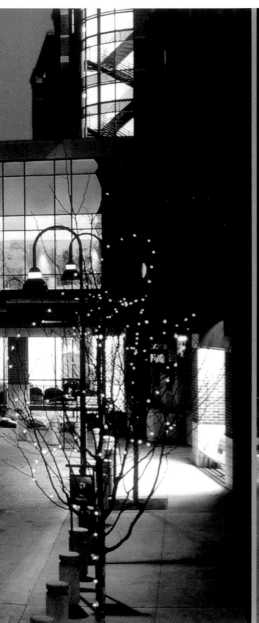
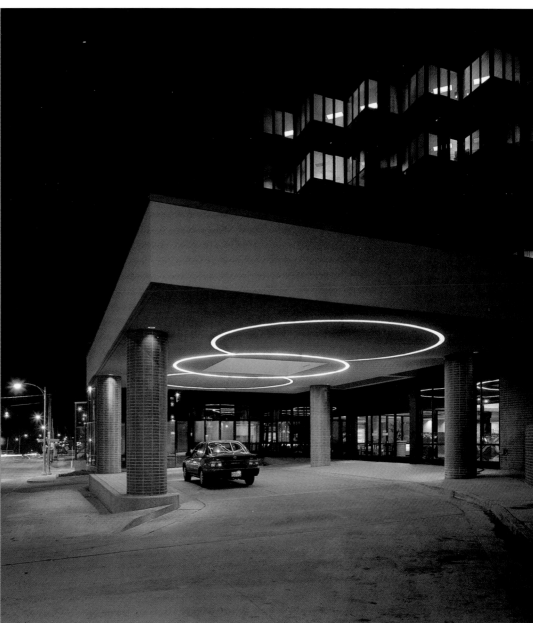

Entrance, Le Bonheur Children's Medical Center, Memphis TN
© Robert Ames Cook

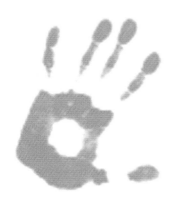
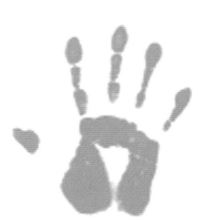

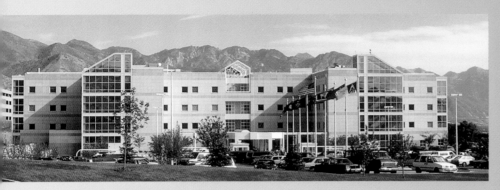

Left, below and right:
Primary Children's Medical Center,
Salt Lake City UT
© Steven Elbert

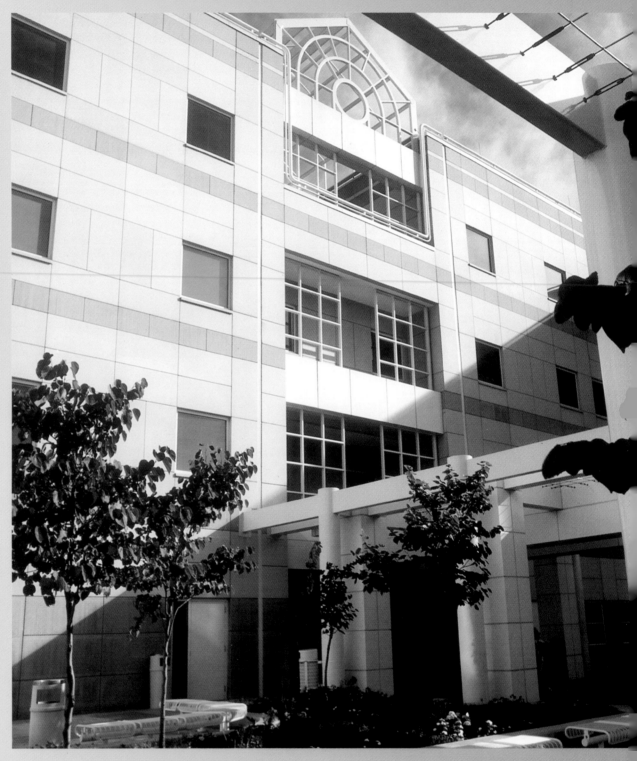

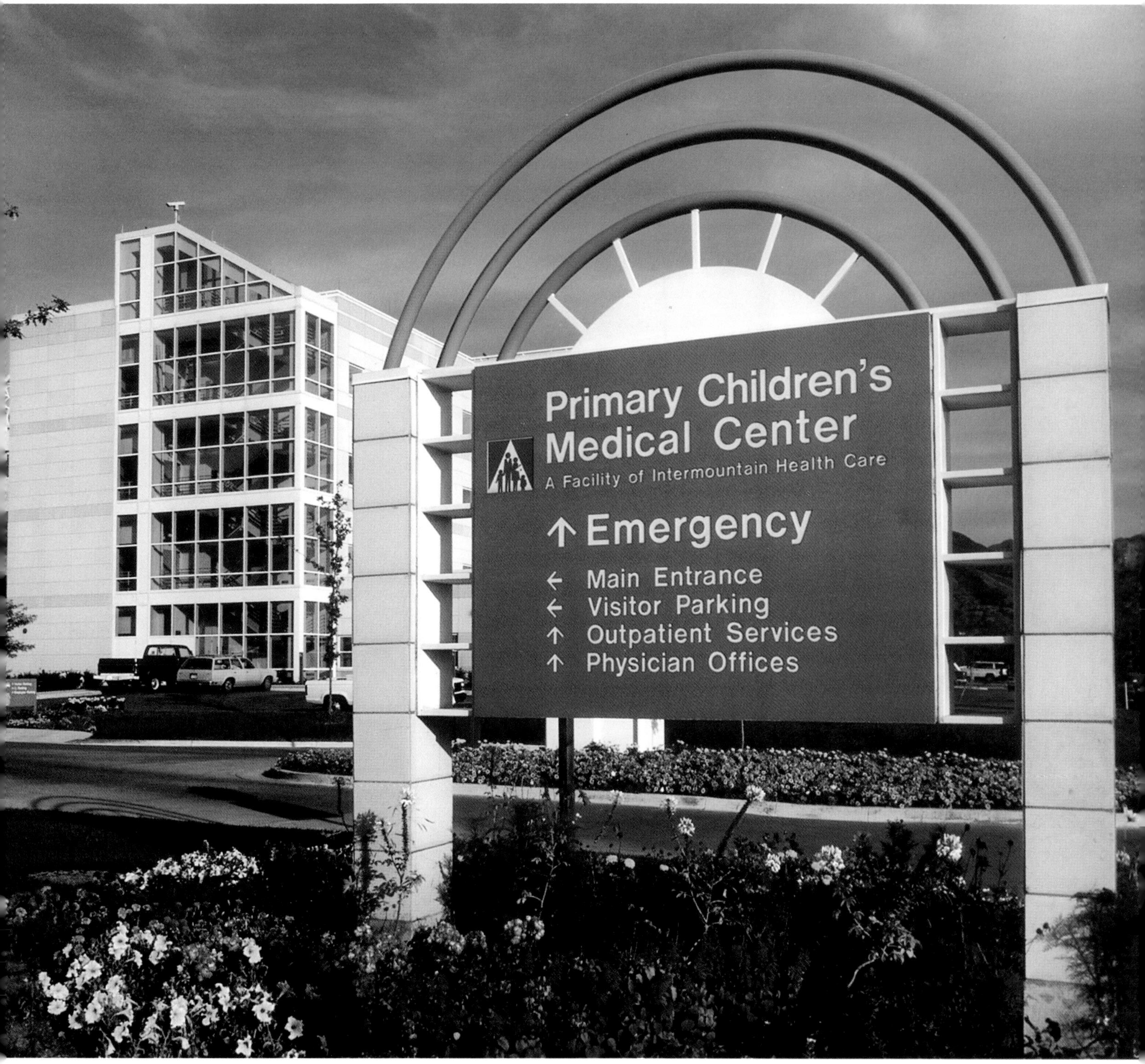
Primary Children's
Medical Center
A Facility of Intermountain Health Care
↑ Emergency
← Main Entrance
← Visitor Parking
↑ Outpatient Services
↑ Physician Offices

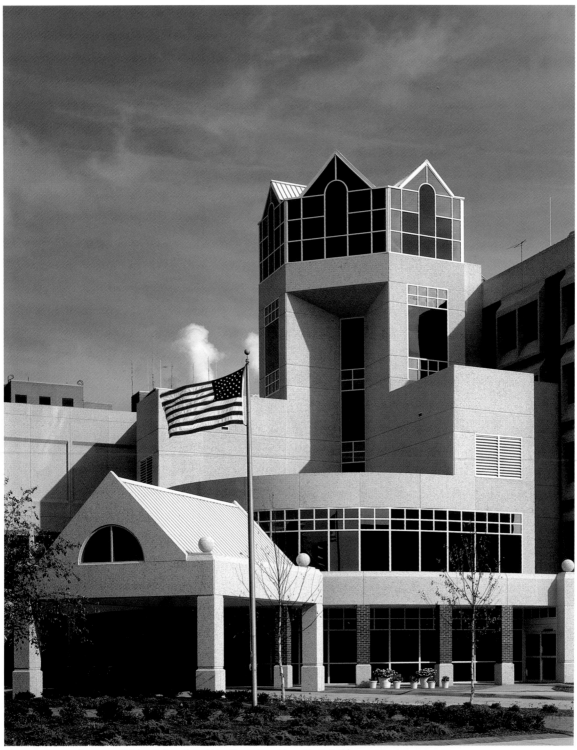

Above and opposite page: Children's Hospital of the King's Daughters, Norfolk VA
© Lisa Masson

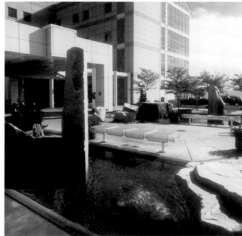

Primary Children's Medical Center, Salt Lake City UT
© Primary Children's Medical Center

20

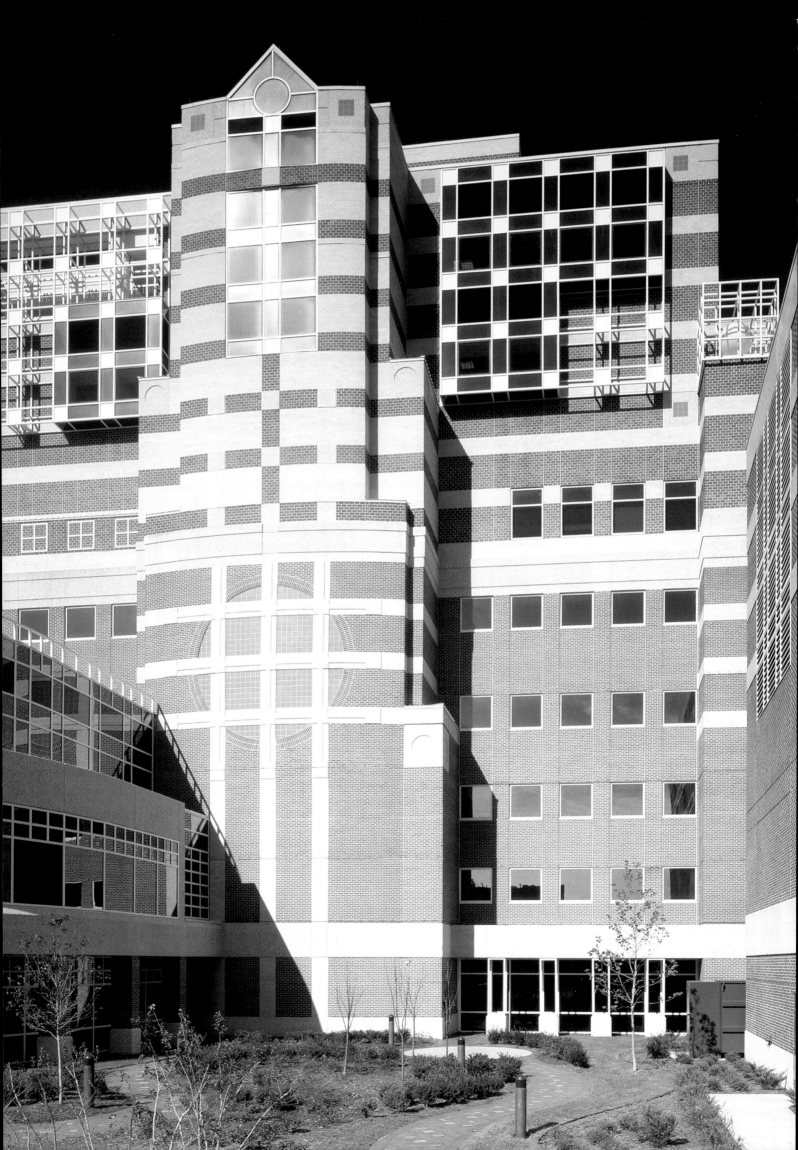

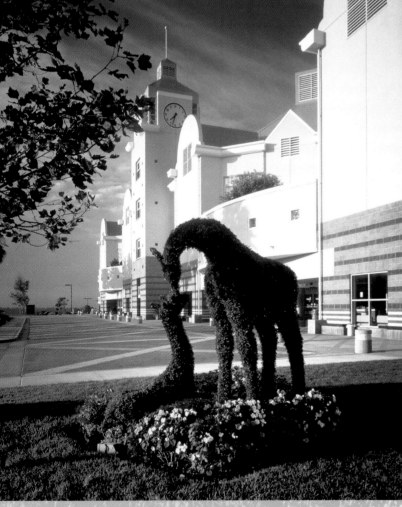

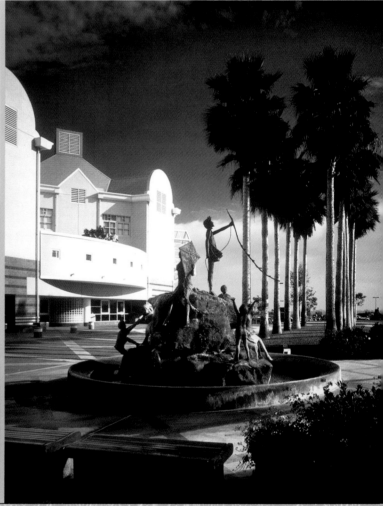

Left and right: Children's Hospital and Health Center, San Diego CA
© Children's Hospital and Health Center

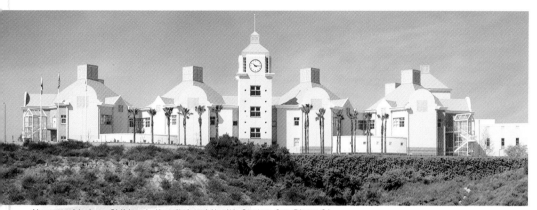

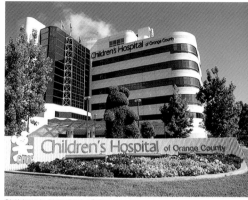

Above and below: Children's Hospital and Health Center, San Diego CA
© David Hewitt/Anne Garrison

Children's Hospital of Orange County,
Orange County CA
© Children's Hospital of Orange County

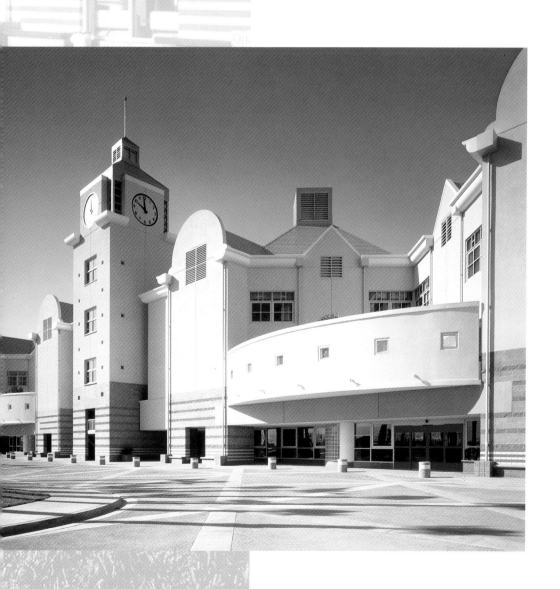

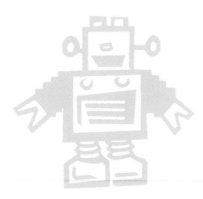

Right and below:
Rainbow Babies, Cleveland OH
© Timothy Hursley

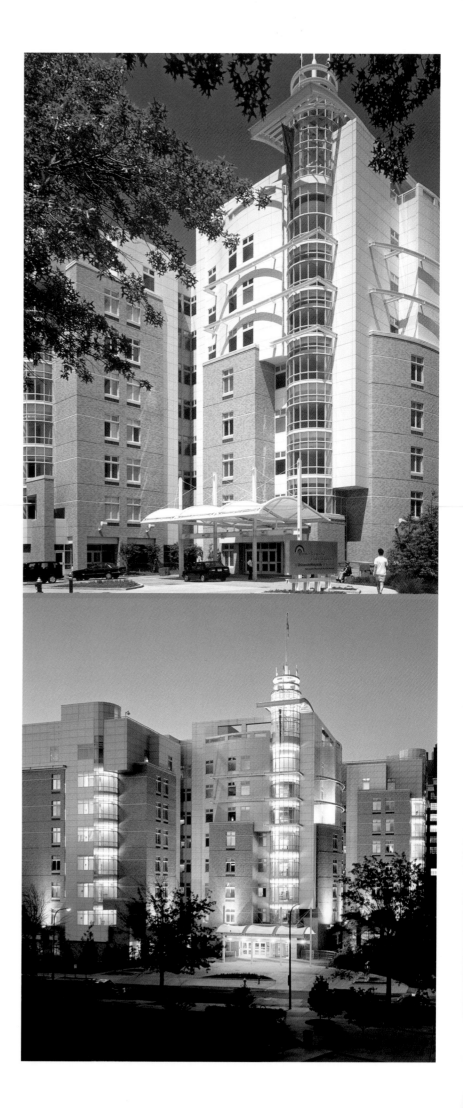

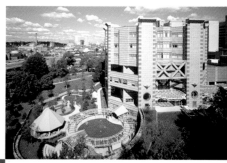

Hasbro Children's Hospital, Providence RI
© Jean Smith

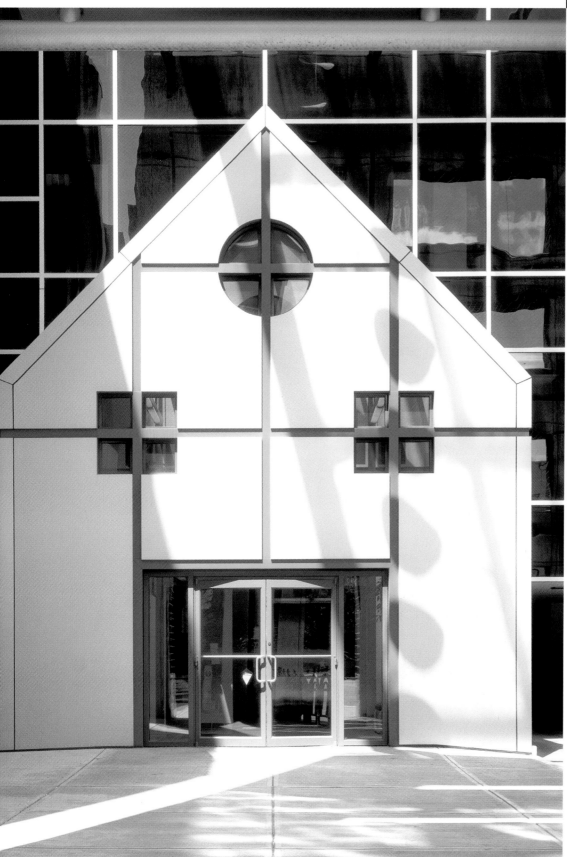

Children's Hospital Medical Center
of Akron, Akron OH
© Children's Hospital Medical
Center of Akron

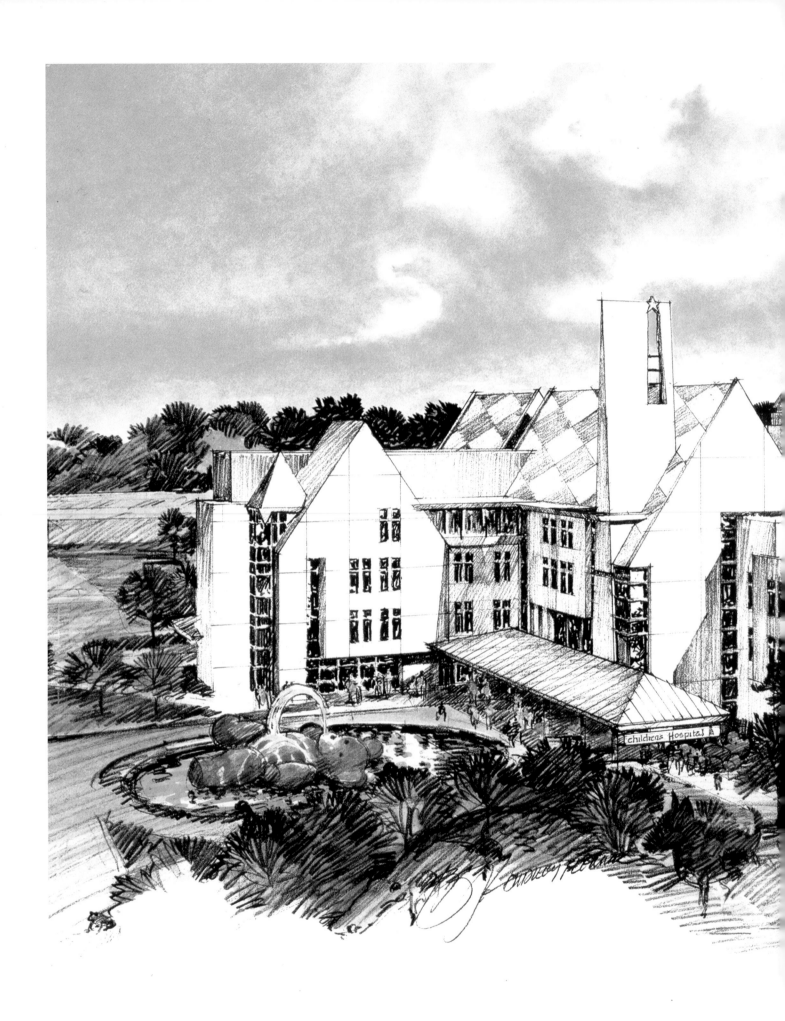

26

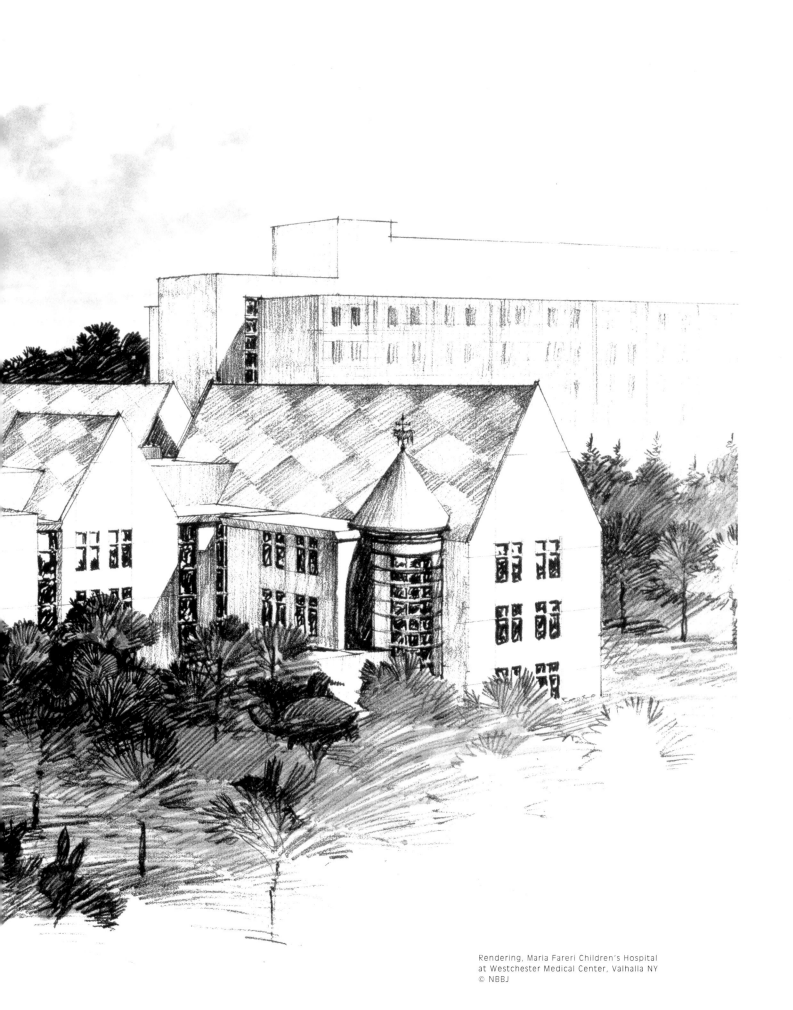

Rendering, Maria Fareri Children's Hospital
at Westchester Medical Center, Valhalla NY
© NBBJ

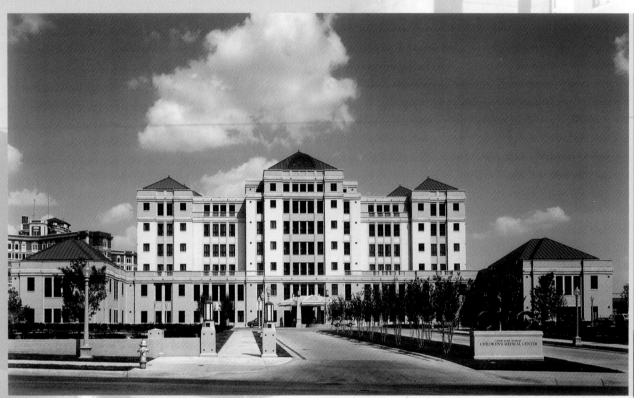

Cook Children's Medical Center, Fort Worth TX
© David M Schwarz/Karlsberger Companies/Architectural Services

Wolfson Children's Hospital, Jacksonville FL
© Wolfson Children's Hospital

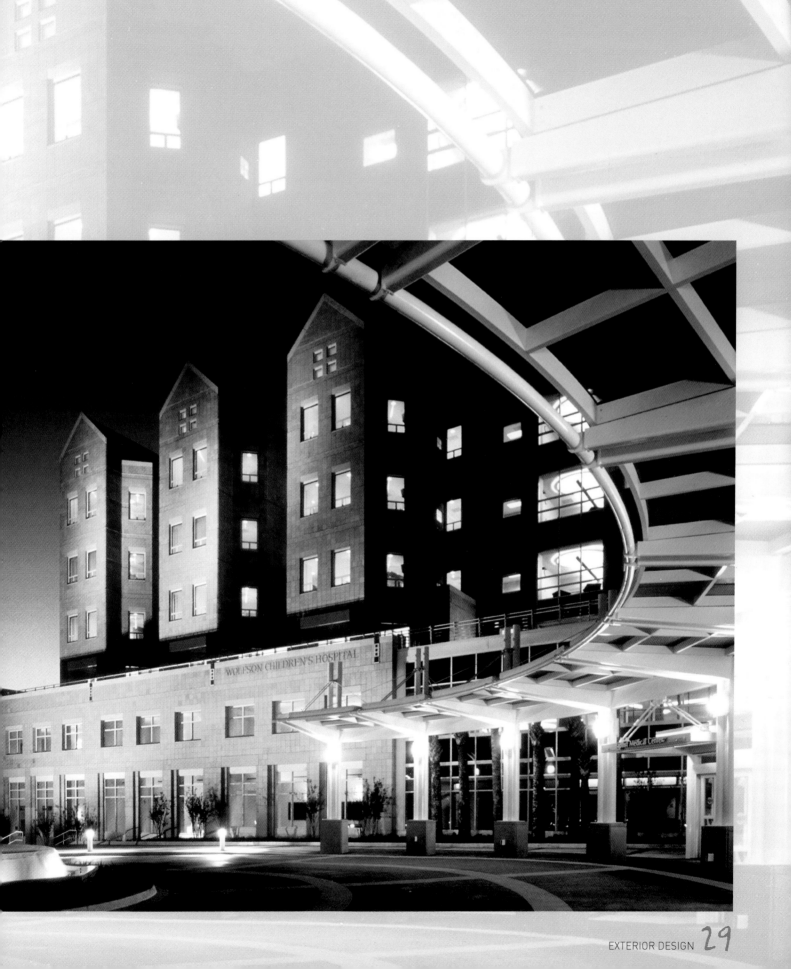

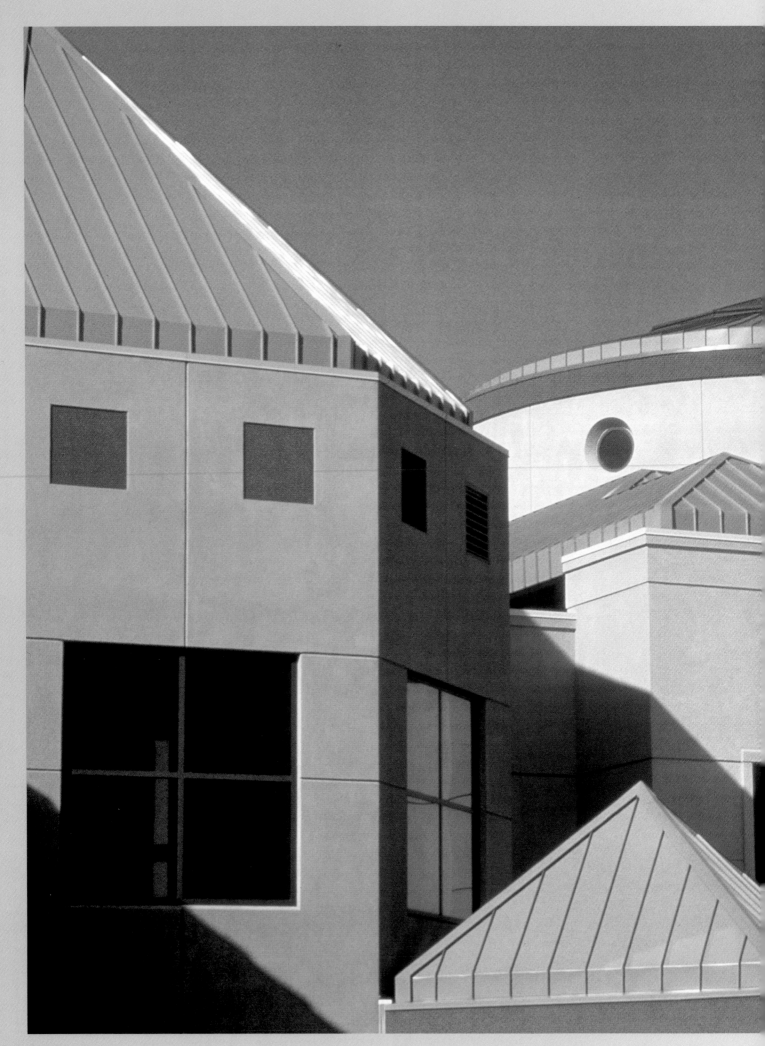

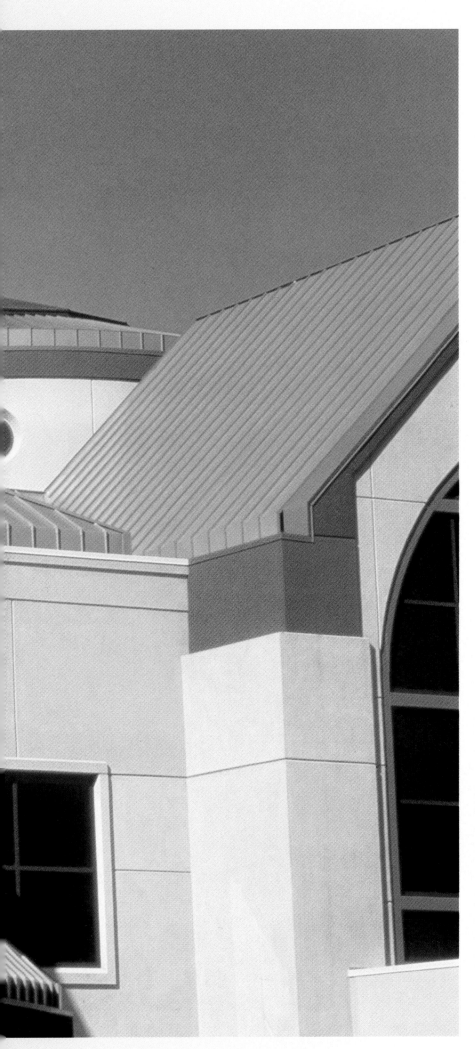

Valley Children's Hospital, Madera CA
© Valley Children's Hospital

Schneider Children's Hospital of Israel, Petach-Tikva, Israel
© Khaled Alkotob

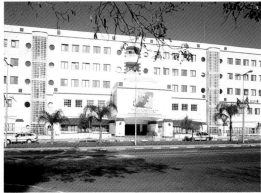

Children's Hospital of Alabama, Birmingham AL
© Children's Hospital of Alabama

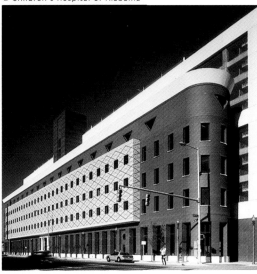

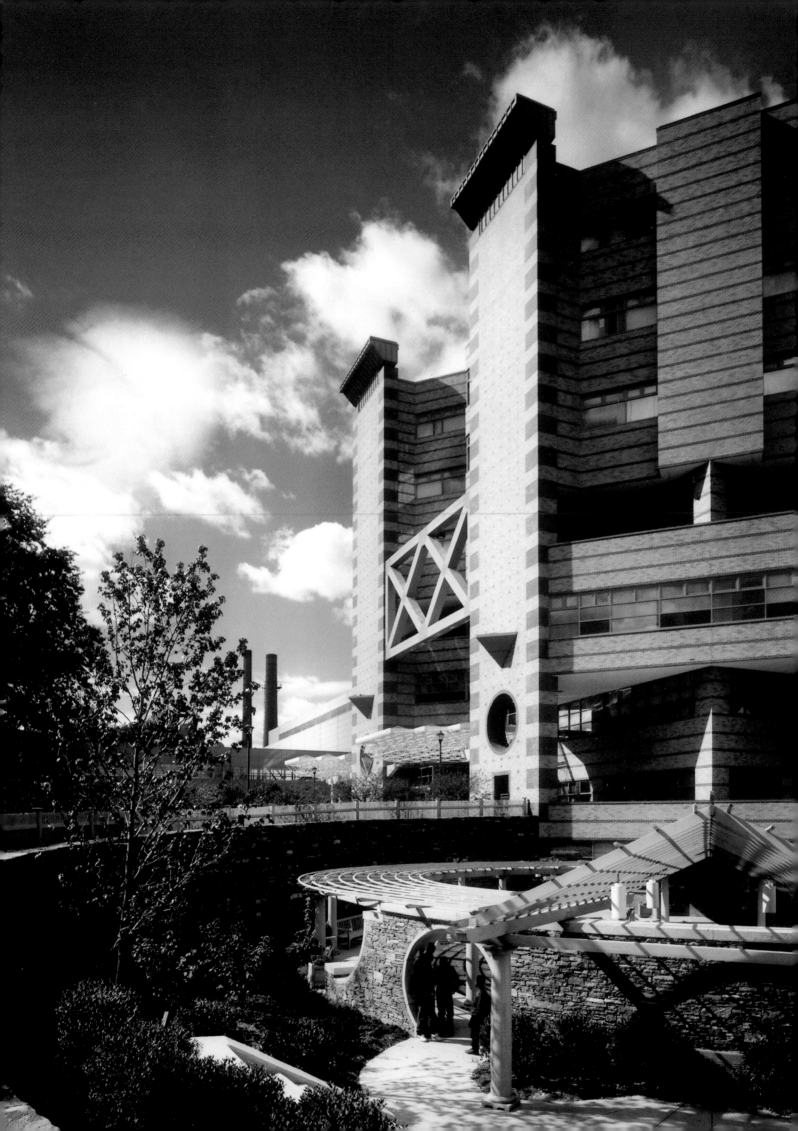

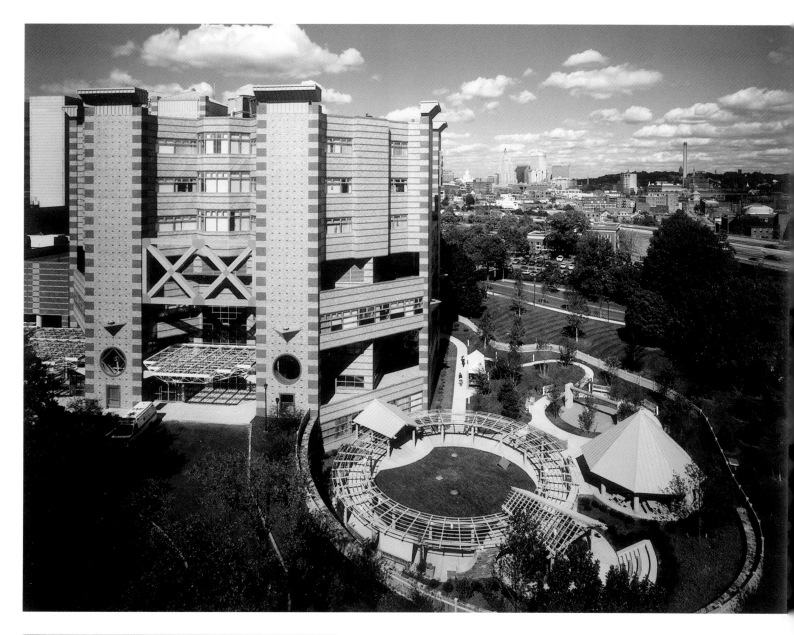

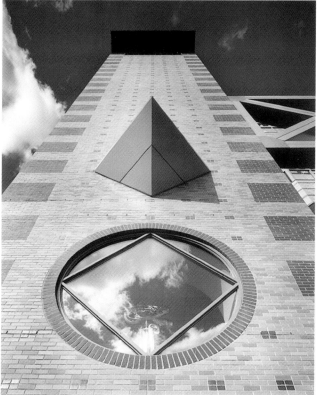

Opposite, above and left:
Hasbro Children's Hospital, Providence RI
© Jean Smith

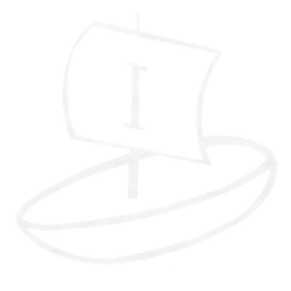

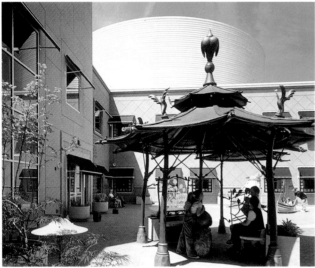

Above and below:
Courtyard, Doernbecher's Children's Hospital, Portland OR
© Timothy Hursley

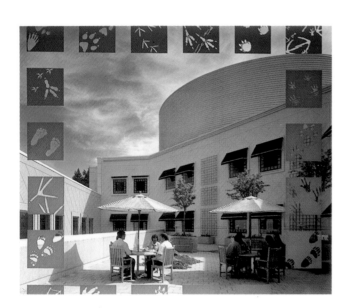

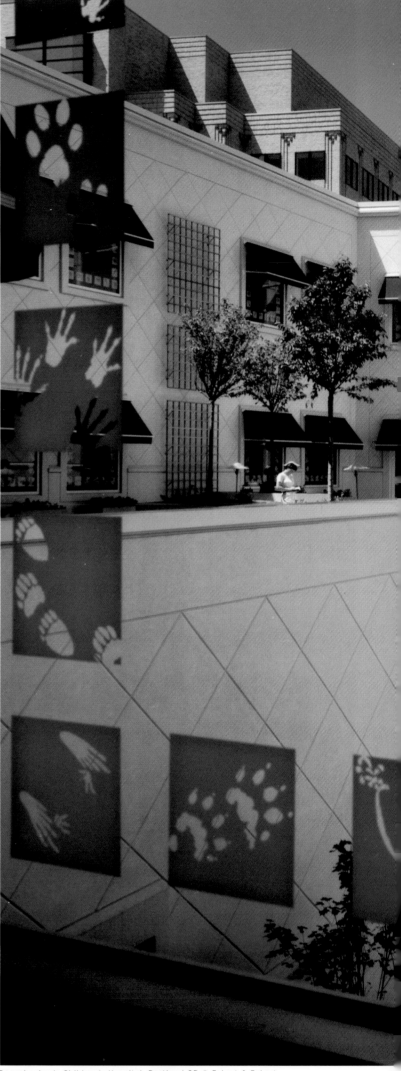

Doernbecher's Children's Hospital, Portland OR © Eckert & Eckert

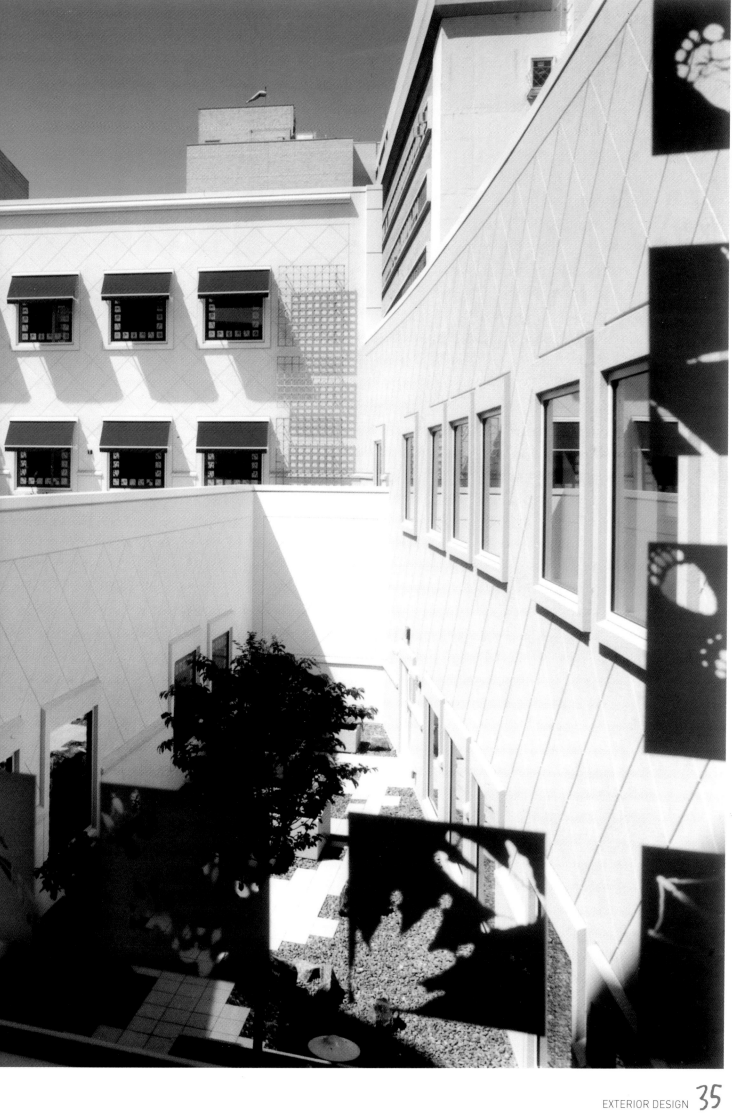

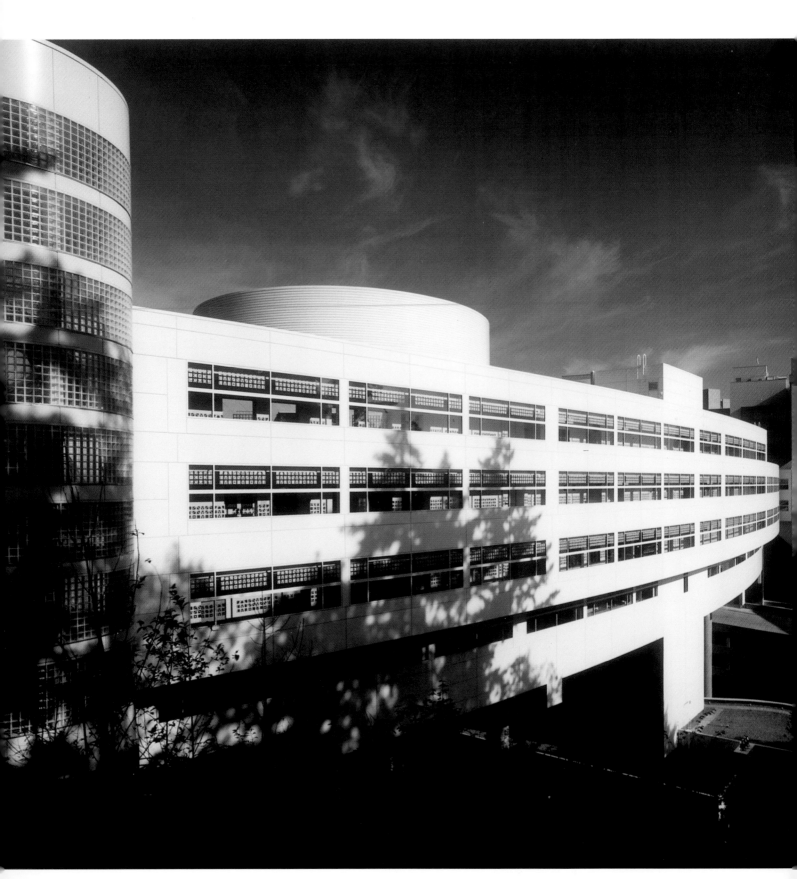

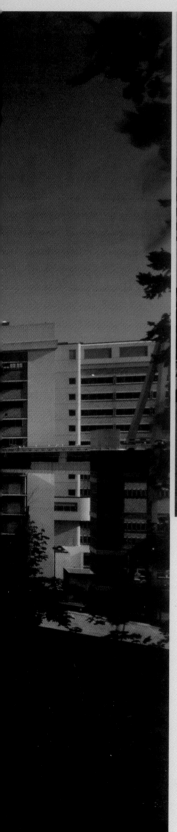

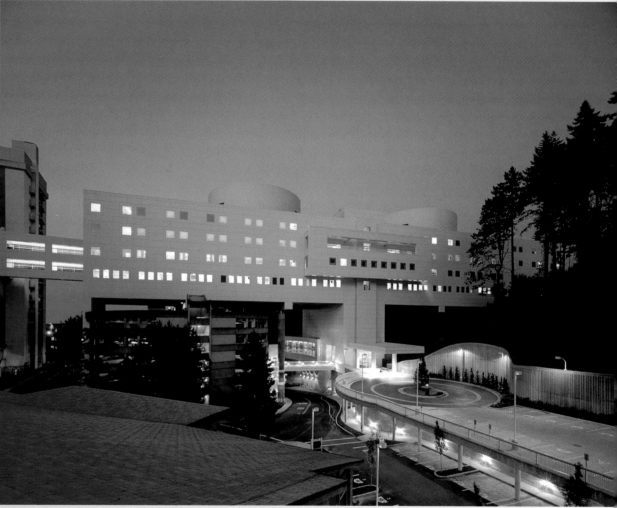

Exterior at night, Doernbecher's Children's Hospital, Portland OR
© Timothy Hursley

Exterior, Doernbecher's Children's Hospital, Portland OR
© Eckert & Eckert

# 2

# Interior Design, Furnishings, & Wayfinding

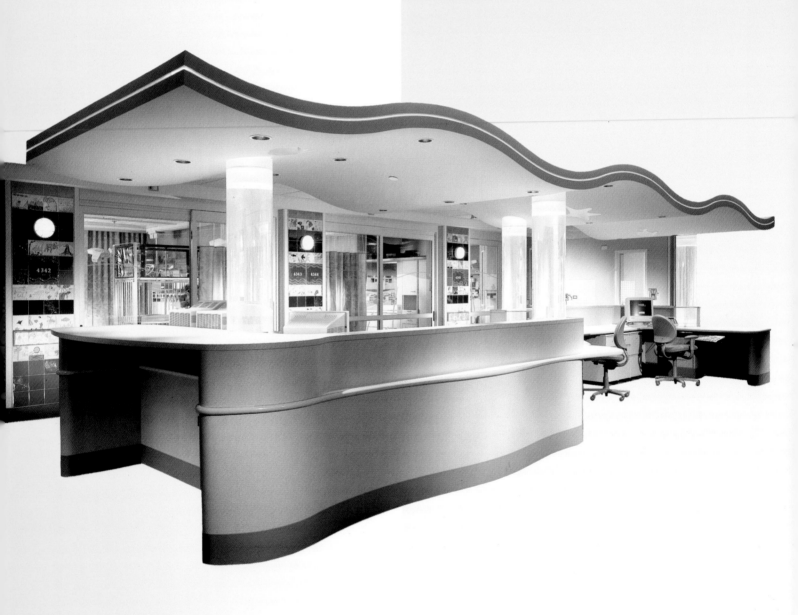

As healthcare becomes increasingly technical and seemingly bureaucratic, the need for a healing environment that offers psychological support is critical. Nowhere is this more keenly felt than in children's hospitals. Interior spaces must be designed for the entire family. The principles of family-centered design provide for ease of movement, comfort, control and understanding.

Positive distractions entertain and reassure children that they are still in control of their environment. Children, regardless of their age, respond to kinetic elements and spaces that encourage interactive play and stimulate the imagination. By encouraging play, design encourages movement and the accompanying wear and tear. Rounded details, durable interior finishes and appropriately scaled furnishings create a safe, yet playful environment.

Daylight, views to nature and the use of full-spectrum color with their positive psychological effects are fundamental components of a healing environment. Light sources animate space to provide a passive, kinetic experience. Access to exterior spaces introduces natural light and views of nature, which provide patients and families with a sense of time and place. The use of full-spectrum color reinforces the healing effect of daylight and allows for the creation of whimsical environments that appeal to children, yet are not childish or condescending to adolescents and adults.

Not only do sick children come in all sizes; they come with parents and siblings. As inpatient units adapt to support a higher acuity of patients, ancillary spaces must flex to serve families' day to day needs. Private spaces, such as family consulting rooms and resource centers, provide comfort, convenience, and sanctuary. Educational and work support spaces provide a continuity of lifestyle during and after the hospital stay. The type and arrangement of furnishings also must support a variety of programmatic requirements.

Few experiences are more disorienting than a hospitalization. Parents need to be able to find critical information and guide their families through the complex web of the healthcare facility. A successful wayfinding system eases anxiety by creating an understandable environment through the use of visual cues and landmarks. Far more than signage, wayfinding systems provide identity and information by integrating the elements of architecture, interior design and art to provide orientation and direction.

Today the interior environment of a children's hospital is for and about children and their families. Spaces are designed to engage the active mind and successfully distract children from the stress related to the anxiety of their visit to the hospital. When children feel comfortable, the family is more relaxed during their stay and the healing process begins. In designing for children's hospitals, we must remember that a child's work is play. The most important thing we do is to provide a child with the opportunity 'to be a child,' especially in a clinical environment.

**John I. Plappert, AIA
and Linda M. Gabel, IIDA**
Karlsberger Companies
Columbus OH

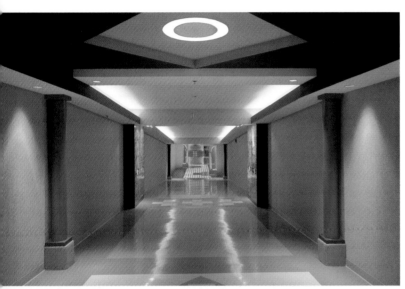

Tunnel, Le Bonheur Children's Medical Center, Memphis TN © Robert Ames Cook

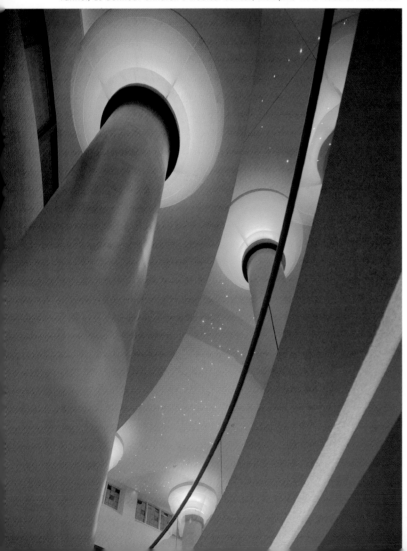

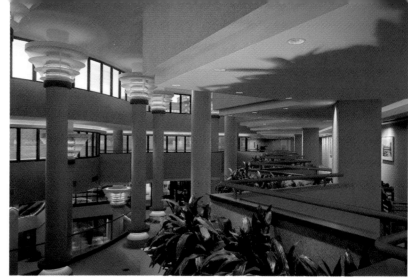

Above, below and bottom left: Lobby, Le Bonheur Children's Medical Center, Memphis TN © Robert Ames Cook

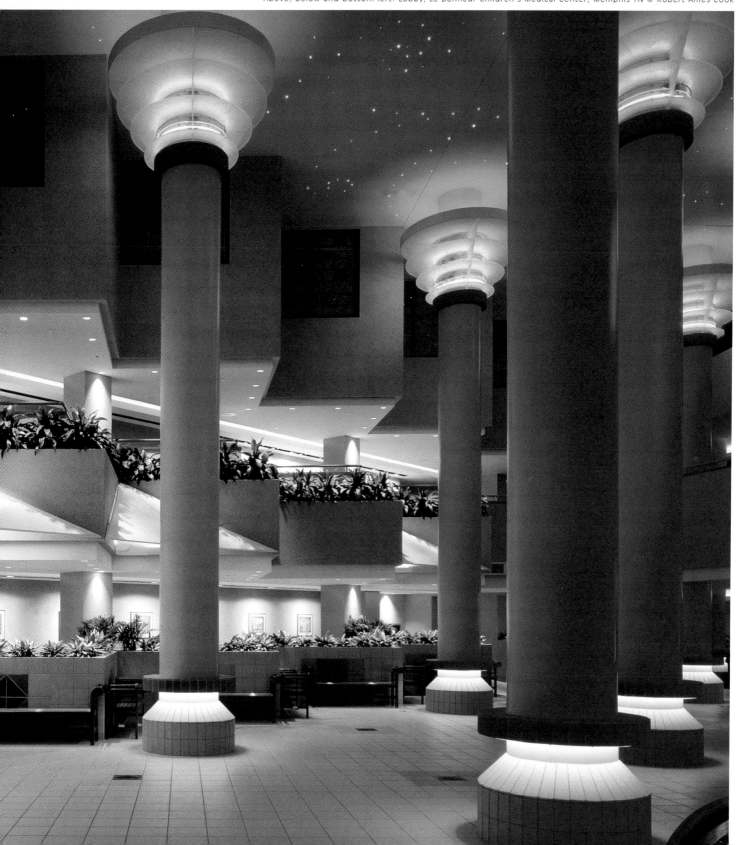

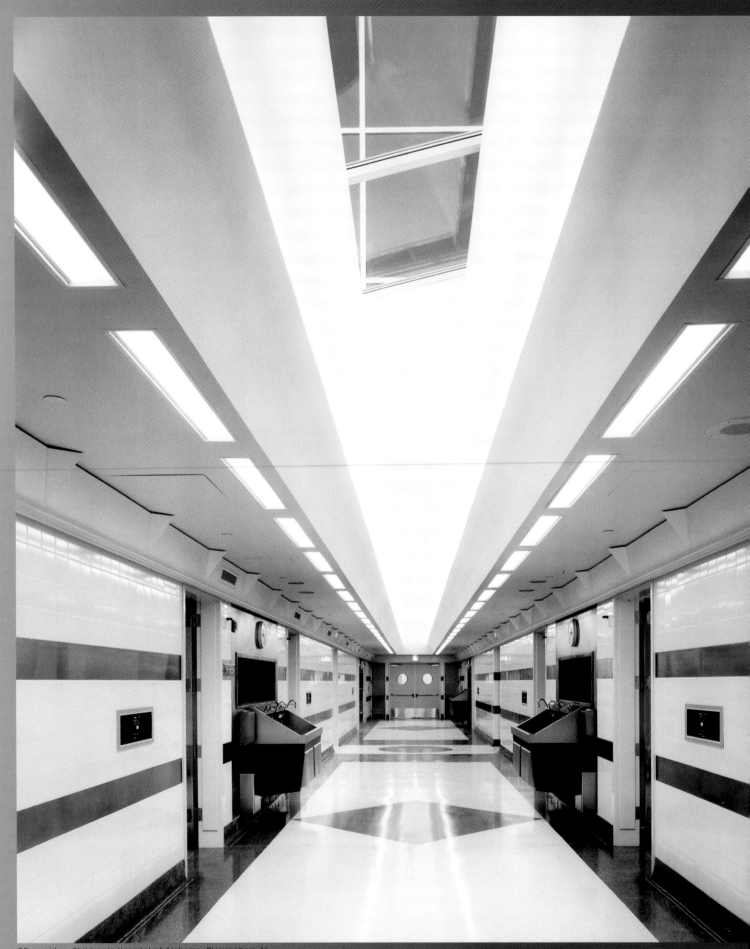

OR corridor, Children's Hospital of Alabama, Birmingham AL
© Children's Hospital of Alabama

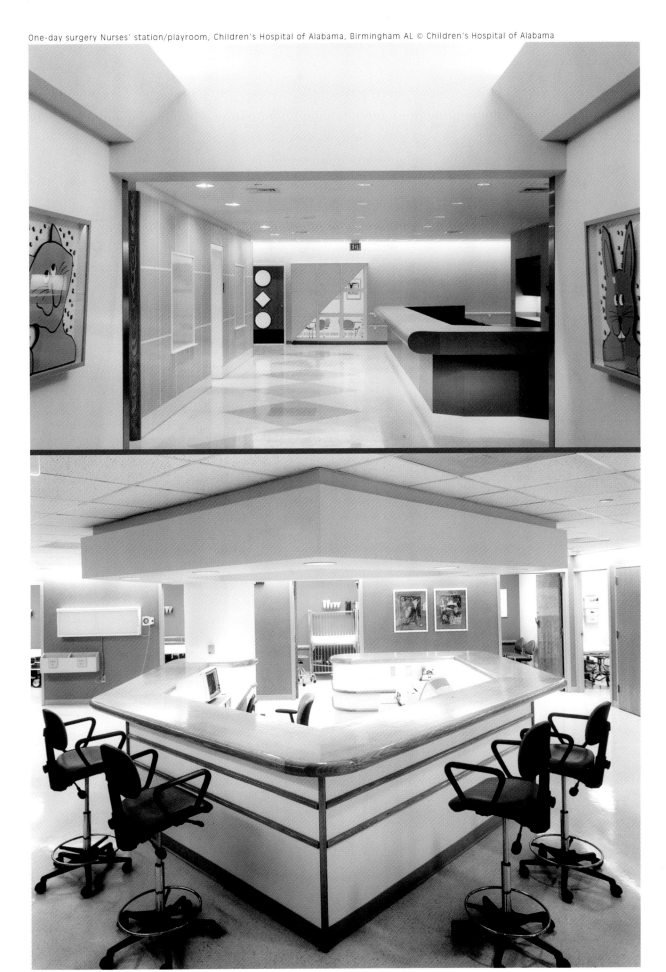

One-day surgery Nurses' station/playroom, Children's Hospital of Alabama, Birmingham AL © Children's Hospital of Alabama

Nurses' station, Children's Hospital of Alabama, Birmingham AL
© Robert Ames Cook

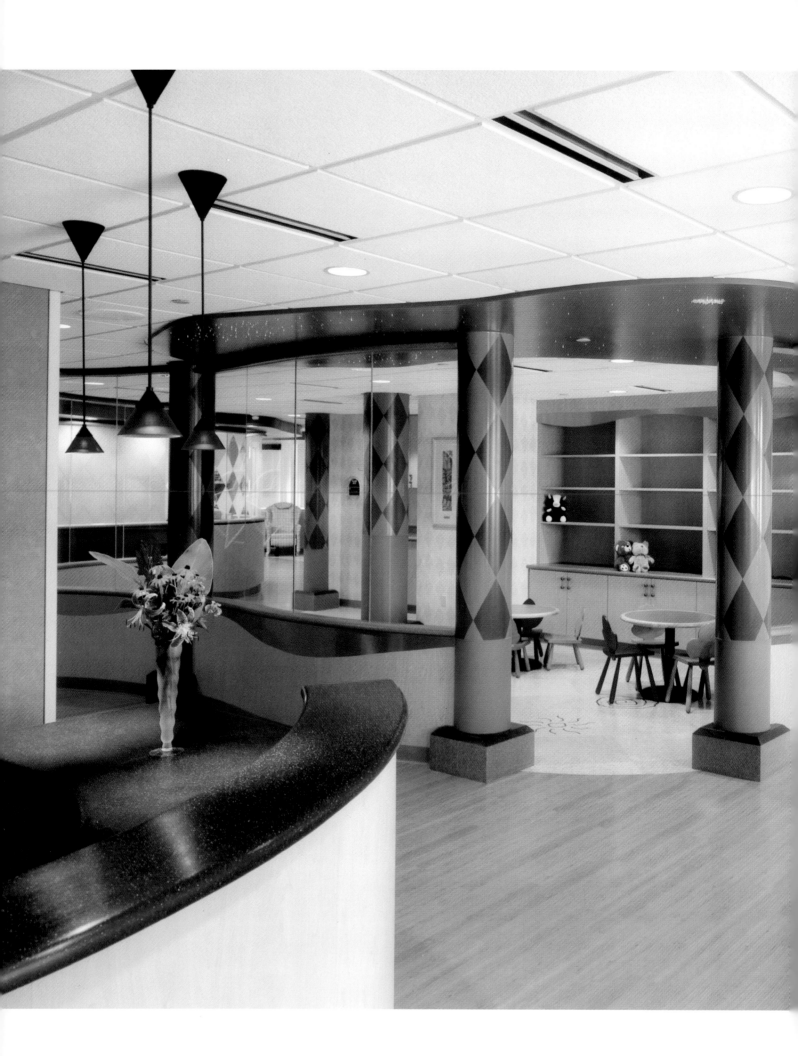

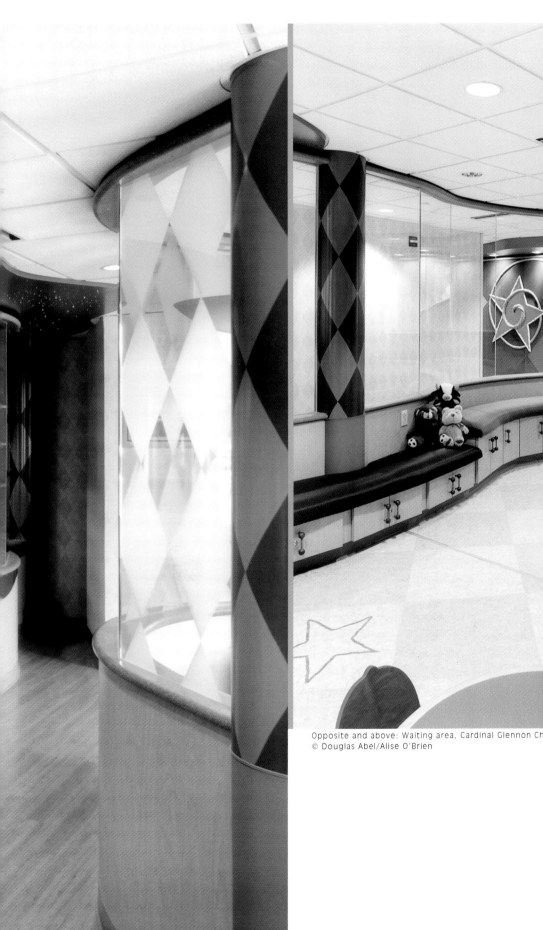

Opposite and above: Waiting area, Cardinal Glennon Children's Hospital, St Louis MO
© Douglas Abel/Alise O'Brien

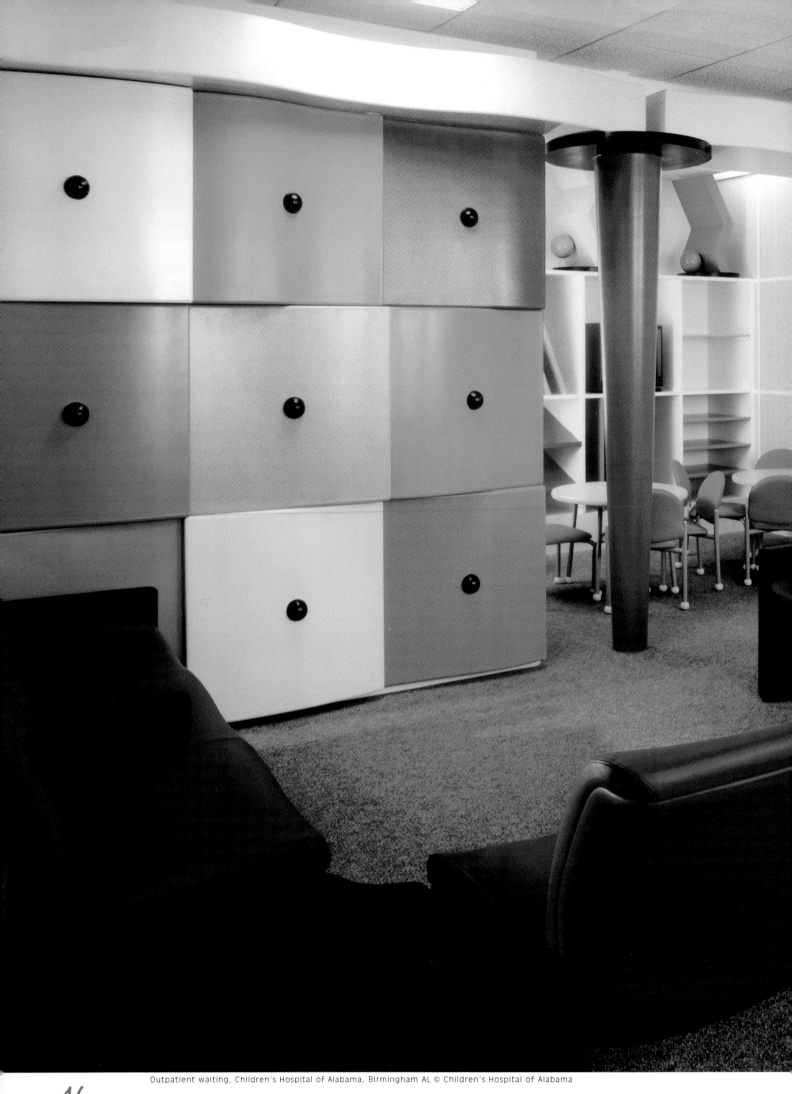

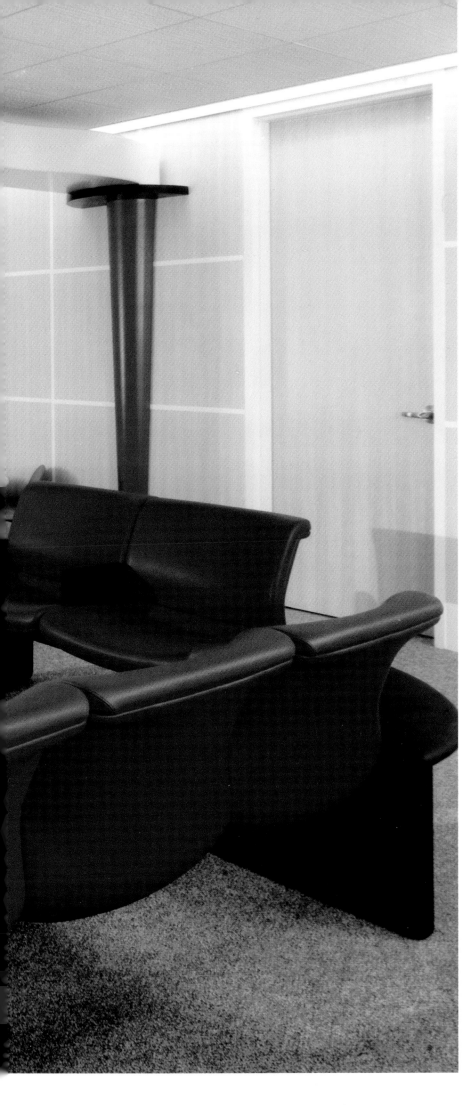

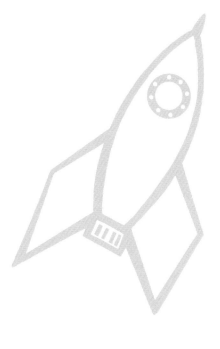

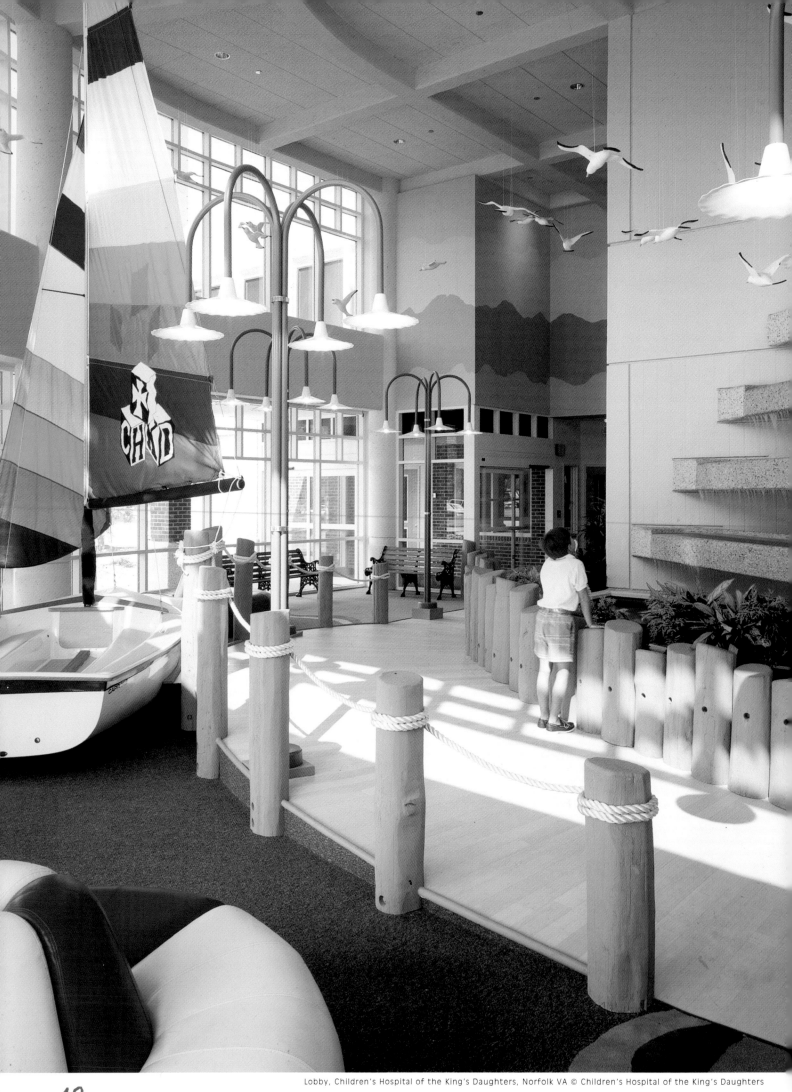

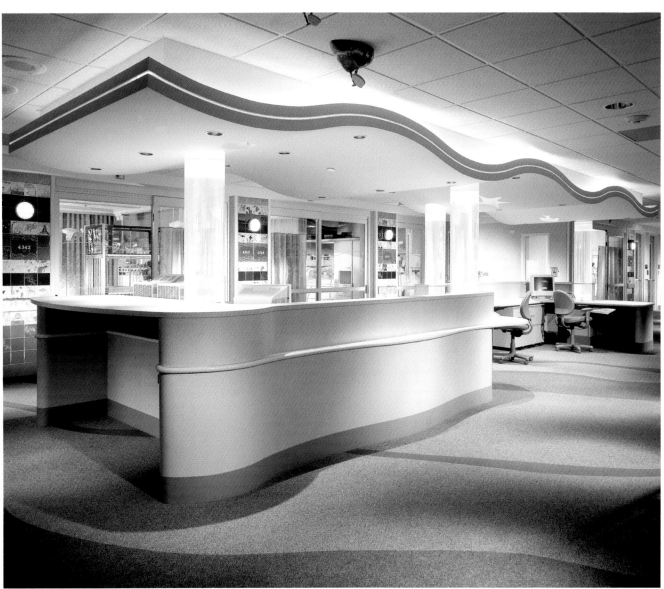

Loyola PICU Nurses' station, Children's Hospital of the King's Daughters, Norfolk VA
© Children's Hospital of the King's Daughters

Loyola PICU hallway, Children's Hospital of the King's Daughters, Norfolk VA
© Children's Hospital of the King's Daughters

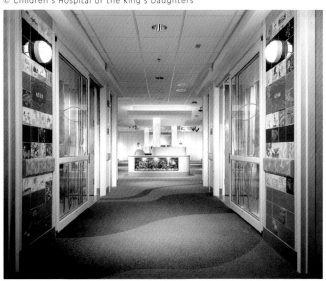

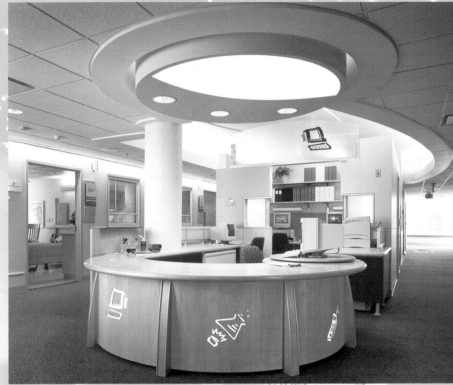

Nurses' station, Rainbow Babies, Cleveland OH © Timothy Hursley

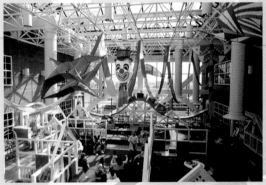

Atrium/playroom, Children's Hospital
University of South Carolina, Charleston SC
© Children's Hospital, University of South Carolina

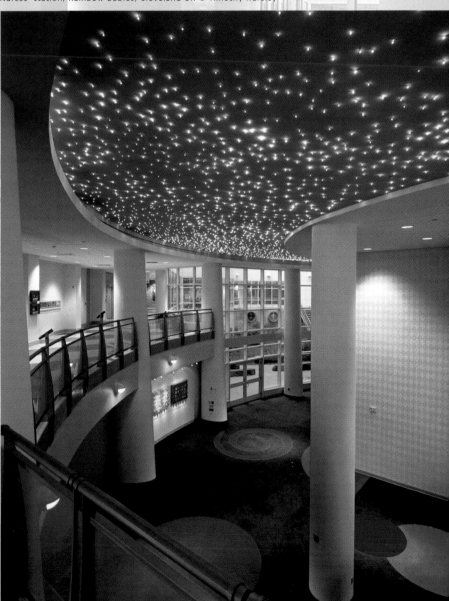

Above and right: Lobby, Rainbow Babies, Cleveland OH © Timothy Hursley

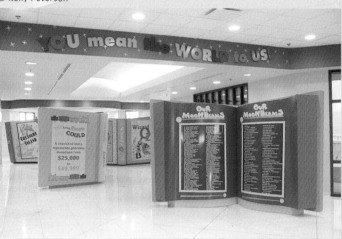

Children's books were designed to highlight various levels
of contribution to Valley Children's Hospital, Madera CA
© Kelly Peterson

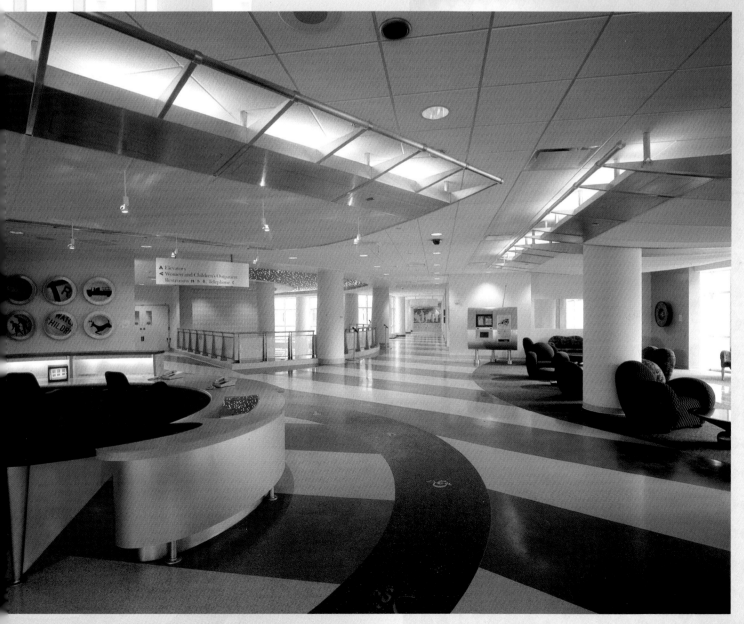

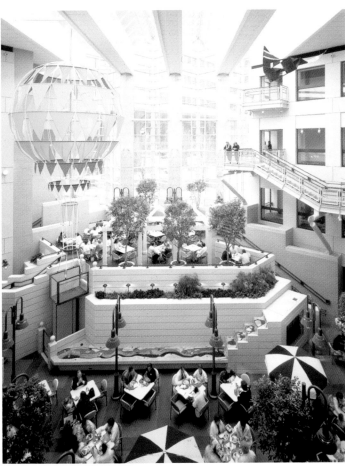

Above and right:
Lobby, St Louis Children's Hospital, St Louis MO
© William E Mathis

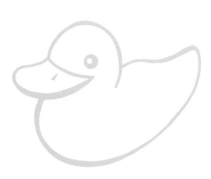

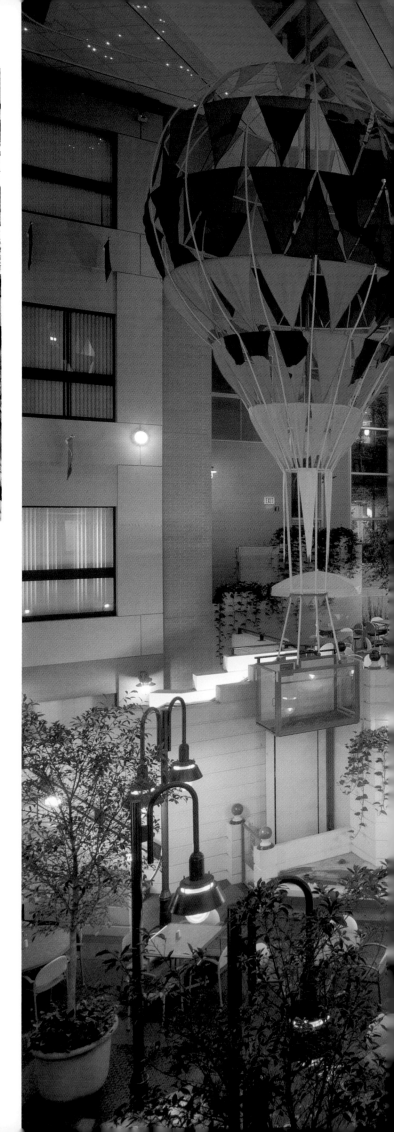

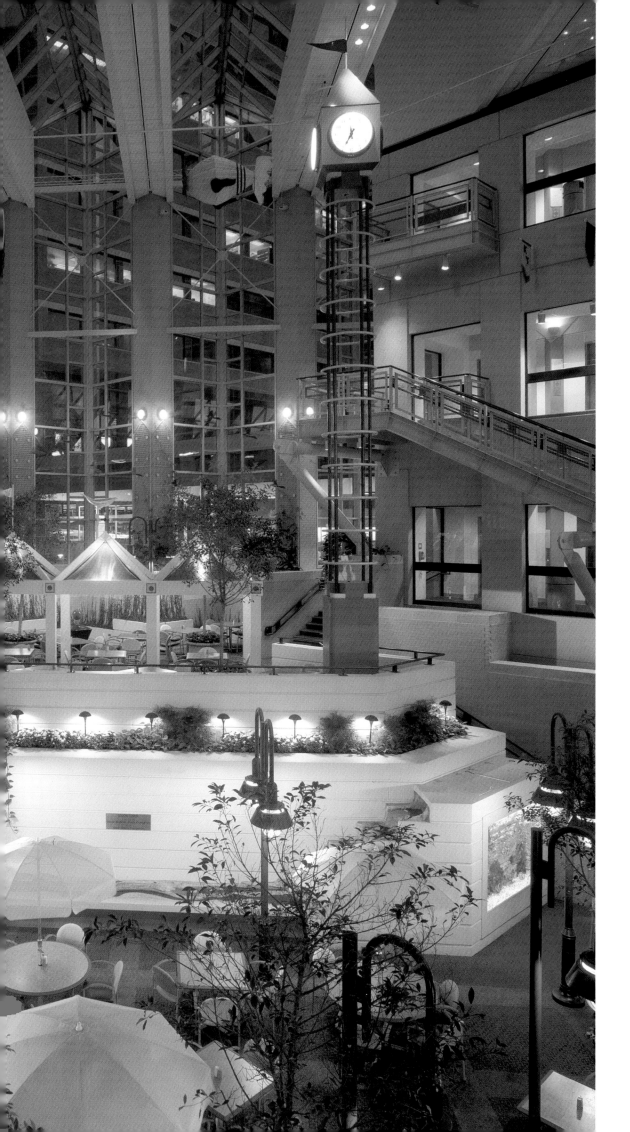

53

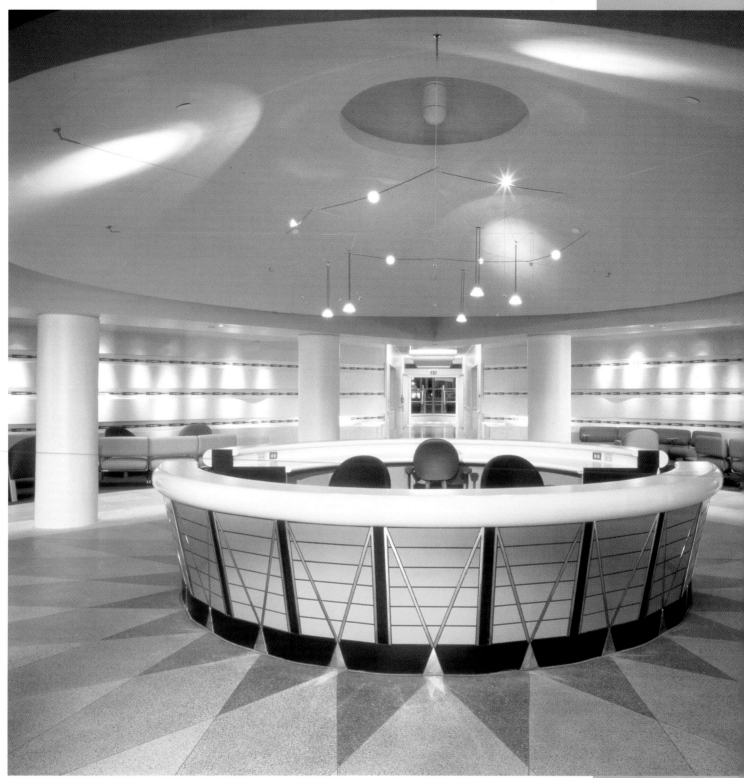

Lobby, Children's Hospital and Health Center, San Diego CA © Children's Hospital and Health Center

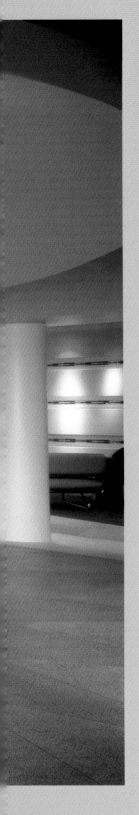

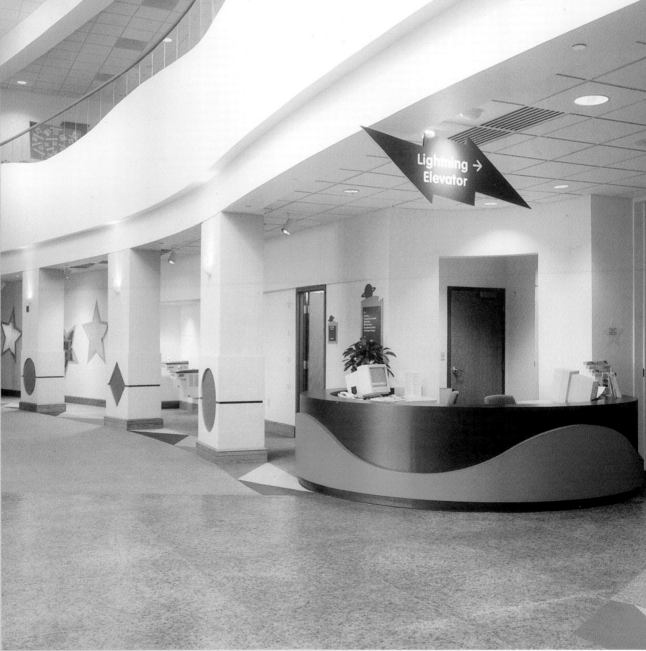

Lobby, Children's Mercy Hospital, Kansas City MO
© Bruce Mathews

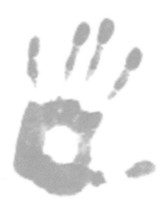

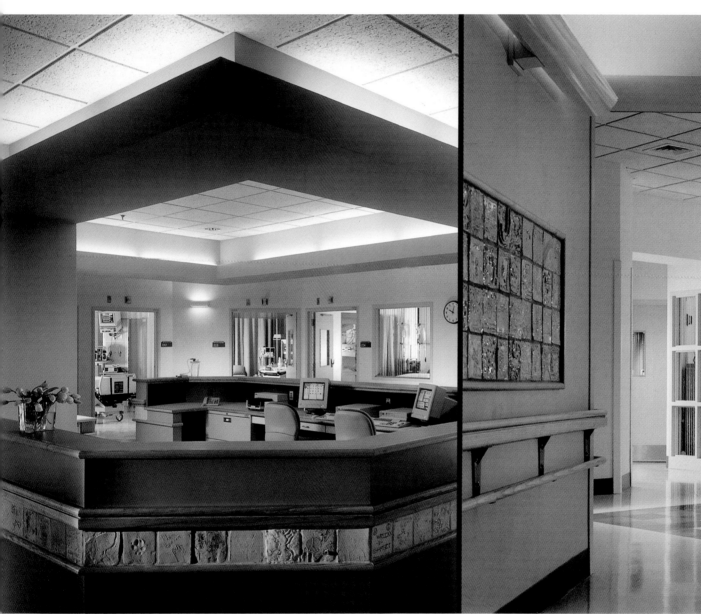

Nurses' station, PICU Hasbro Children's Hospital, Providence RI
© Robert Miller

Family waiting room, Hasbro Children's Hospital, Providence RI
© Robert Miller

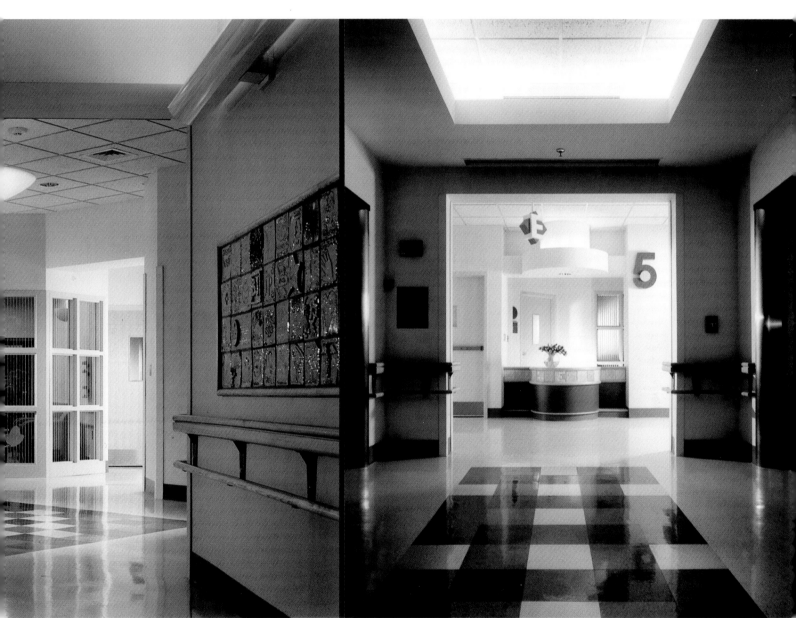

Elevator lobby, Hasbro Children's Hospital, Providence RI
© Robert Miller

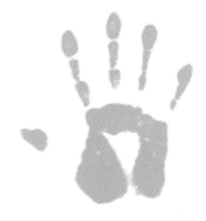

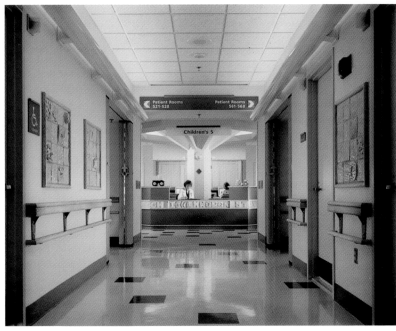

Nurses' station, Hasbro Children's Hospital, Providence RI
© Robert Miller

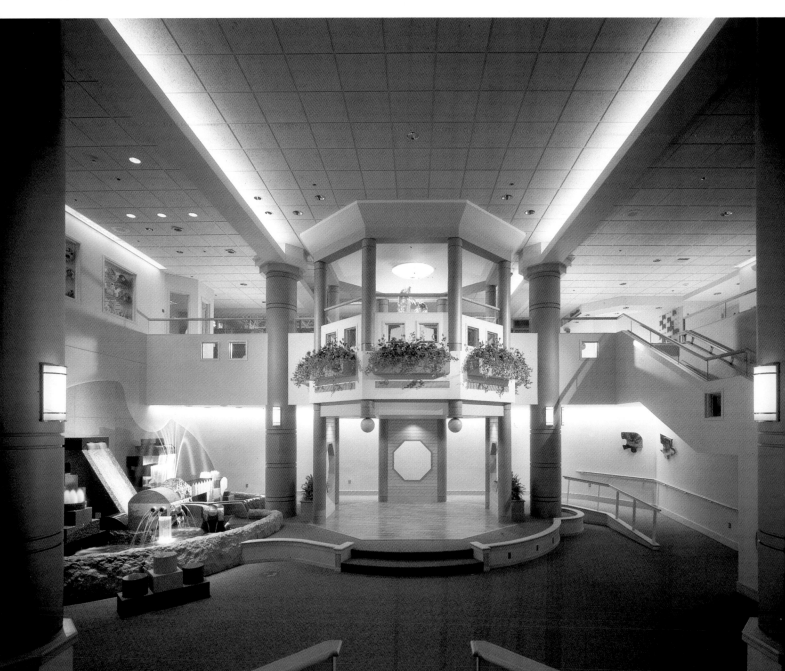

Lobby, Hasbro Children's Hospital, Providence RI
© Robert Miller

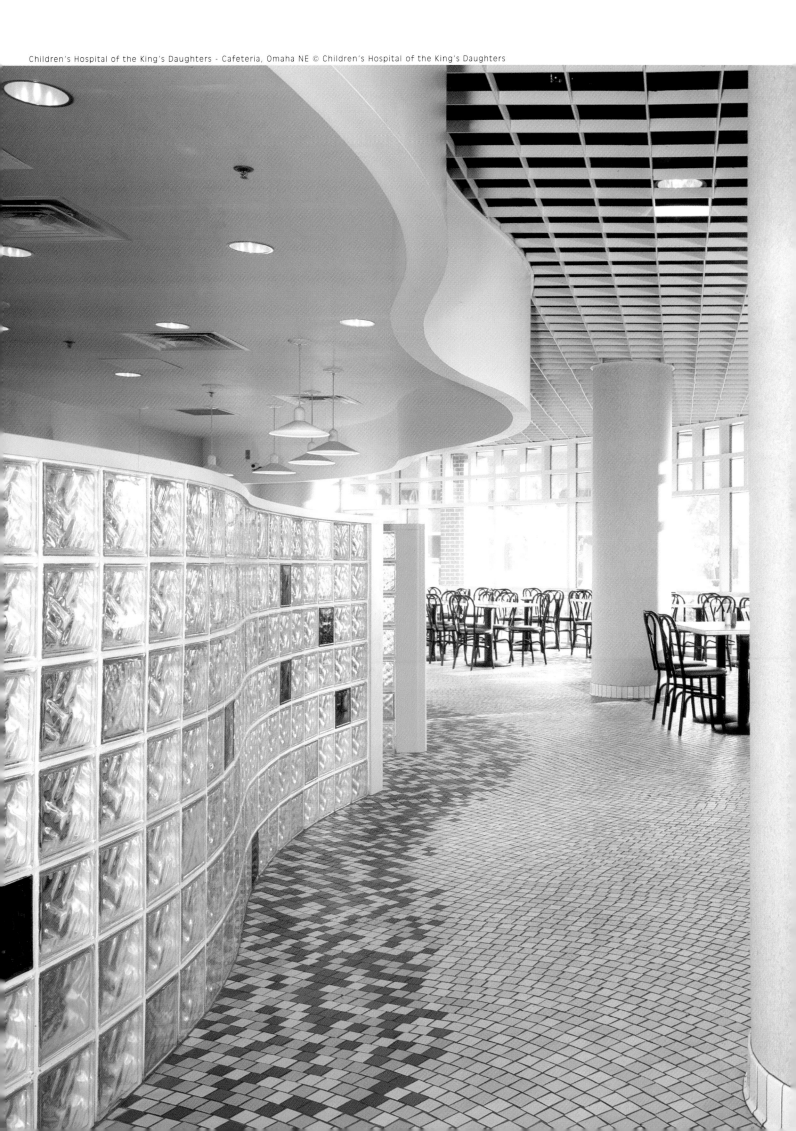

Children's Hospital of the King's Daughters - Cafeteria, Omaha NE © Children's Hospital of the King's Daughters

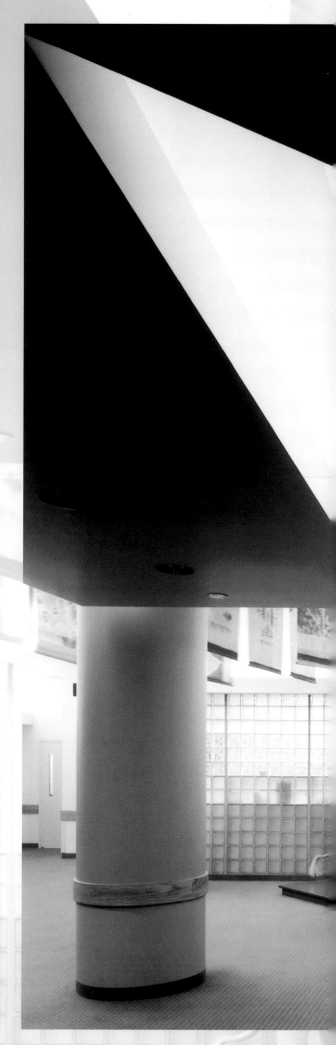

Below and right:
Lobby, Boston Children's Hospital, Boston MA
© Nick Wheeler/Wheeler Photographics

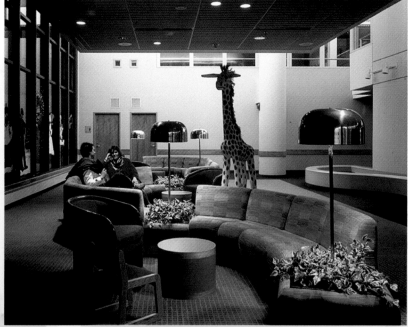

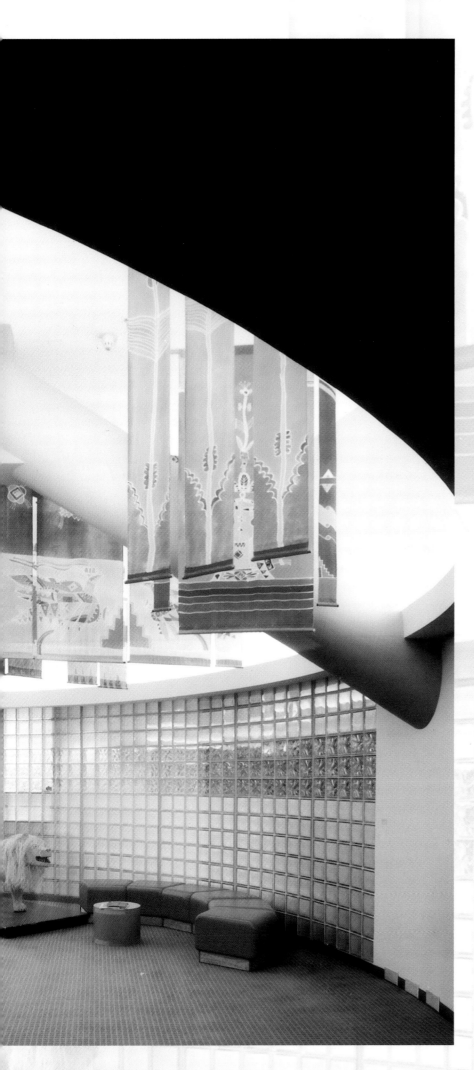

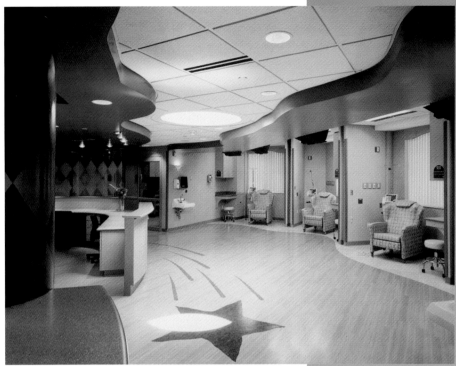

Interior bone marrow treatment area, Cardinal Glennon Children's Hospital, St Louis MO
© Alise O'Brien

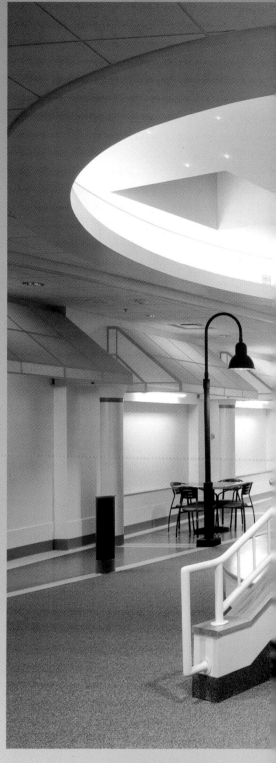

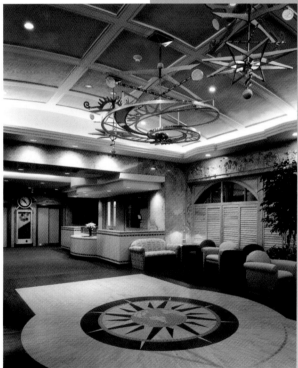

Lobby, Cardinal Glennon Children's Hospital, St Louis MO © Alise O'Brien

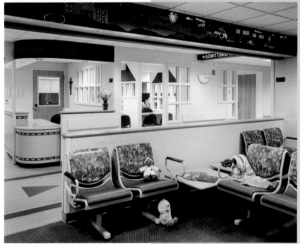

Admitting waiting area, Cardinal Glennon Children's Hospital, St Louis MO © Alise O'Brien

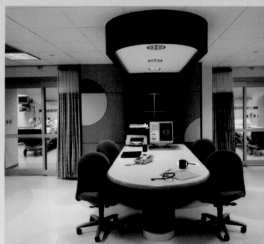

Bone marrow Nurses' station, Cardinal Glennon Children's Hospital, St Louis MO © Alise O'Brien

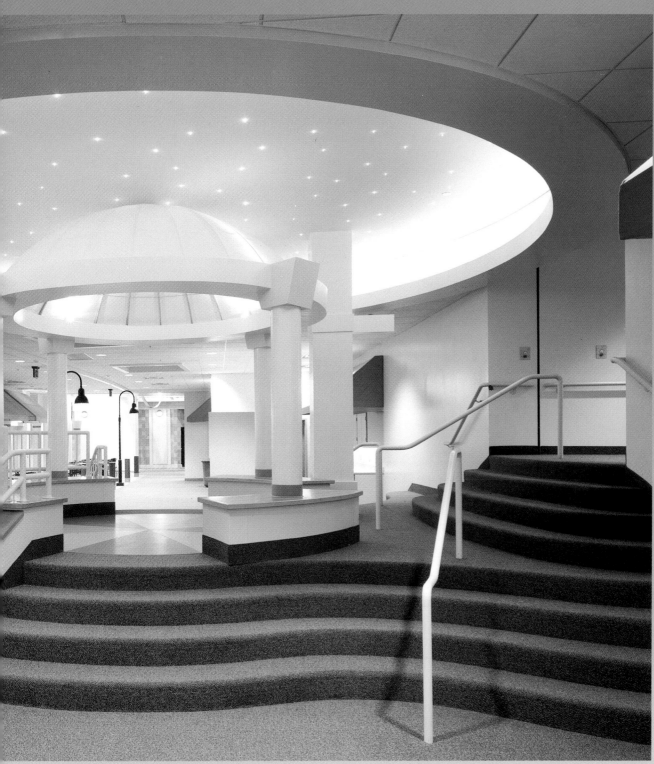

Ambularoty Center lobby, Children's Hospital, Columbus OH
© Children's Hospital

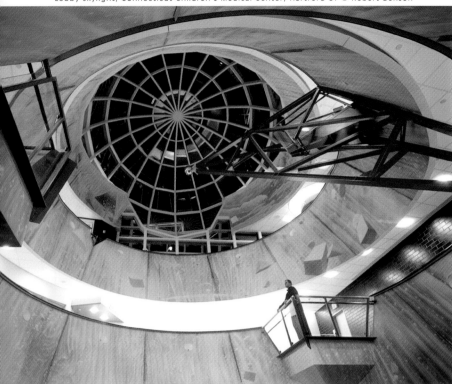

Lobby skylight, Connecticut Children's Medical Center, Hartford CT © Robert Benson

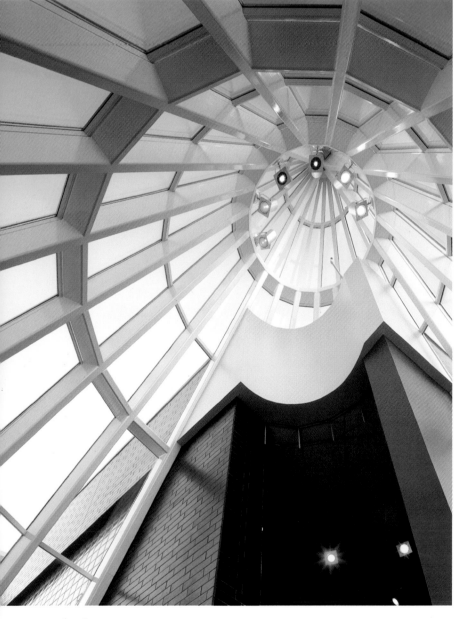

ED skylight, Connecticut Children's Medical Center, Hartford CT © Robert Benson

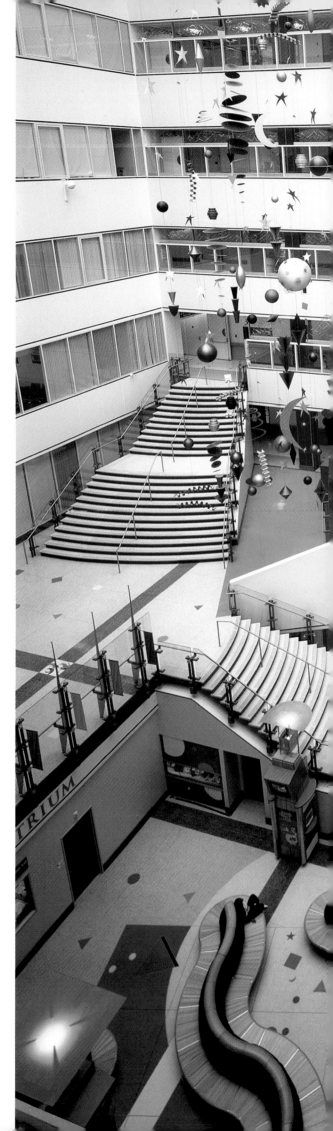

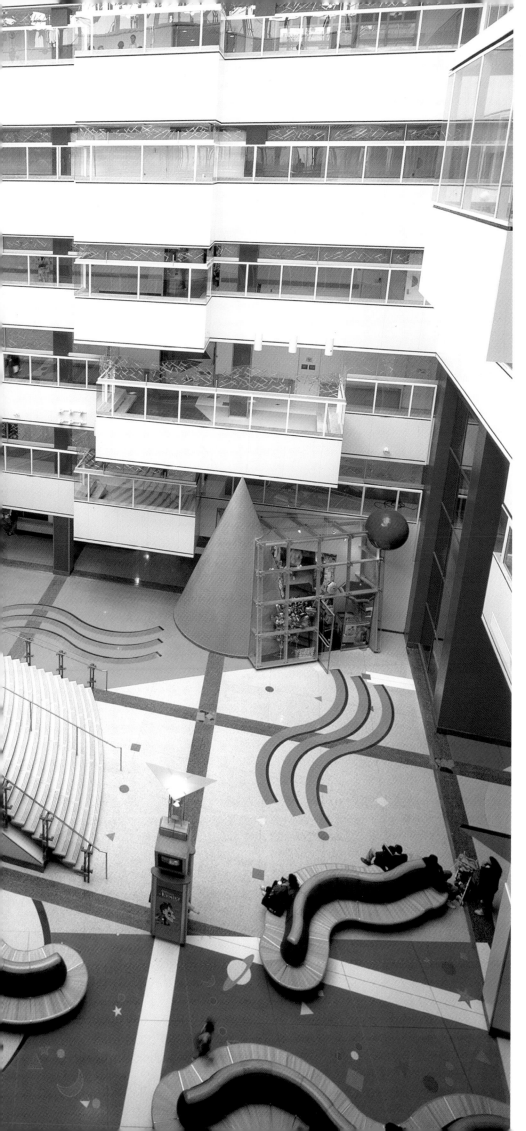

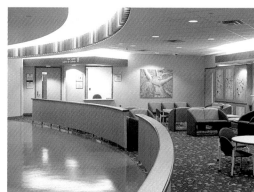

Waiting area, Connecticut Children's
Medical Center, Hartford CT
© Robert Benson

Atrium, The Children's Hospital of Philadelphia,
Philadelphia PA
© Robert Benson

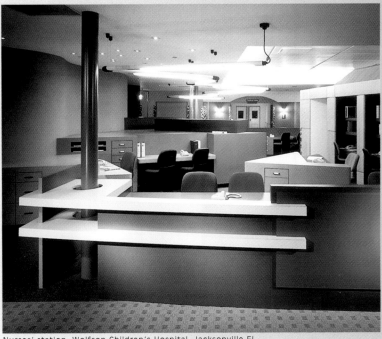

Nurses' station, Wolfson Children's Hospital, Jacksonville FL

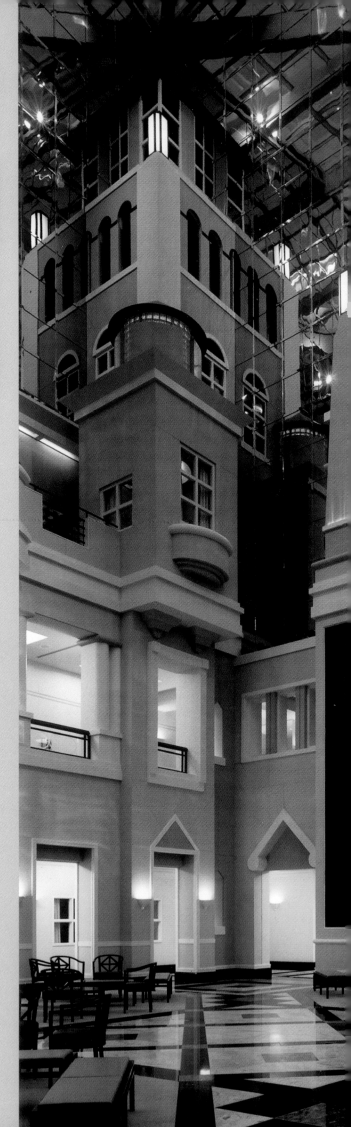

Cook Children's Medical Center, Fort Worth TX © Hedrich-Blessing

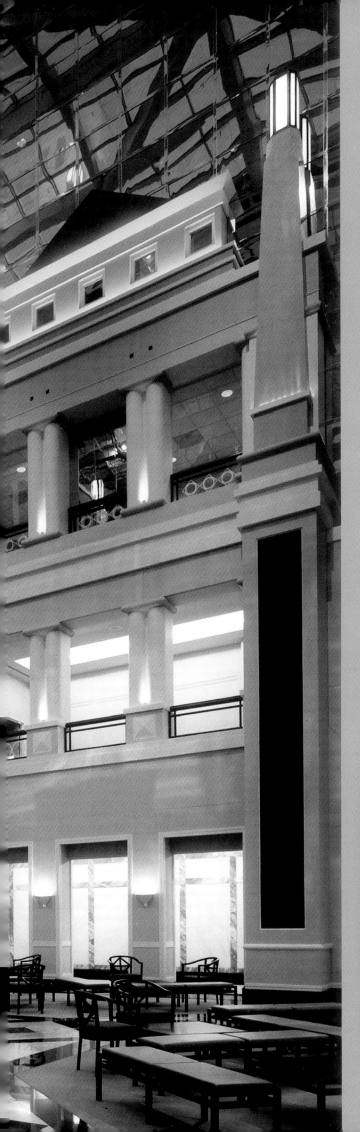

Waiting PICU, Babies & Children's Hospital at New York Presbyterian, New York NY
© Colin McRae

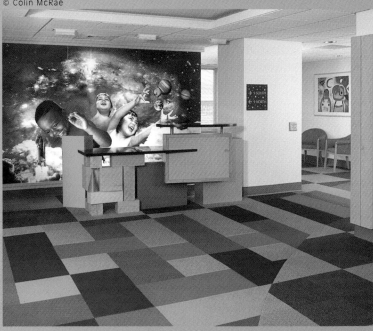

Waiting room, Valley Children's Hospital, Madera CA
© Kelly Peterson

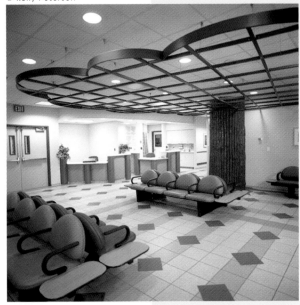

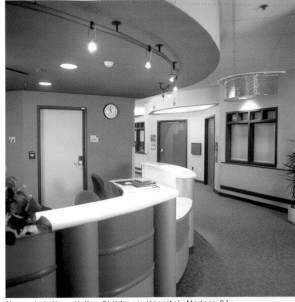

Nurses' station, Valley Children's Hospital, Madera CA
© Kelly Peterson

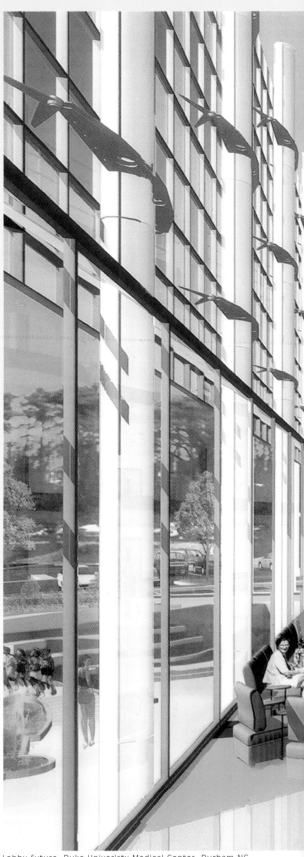

Lobby future, Duke Univeristy Medical Center, Durham NC
© Duke Univeristy Medical Center

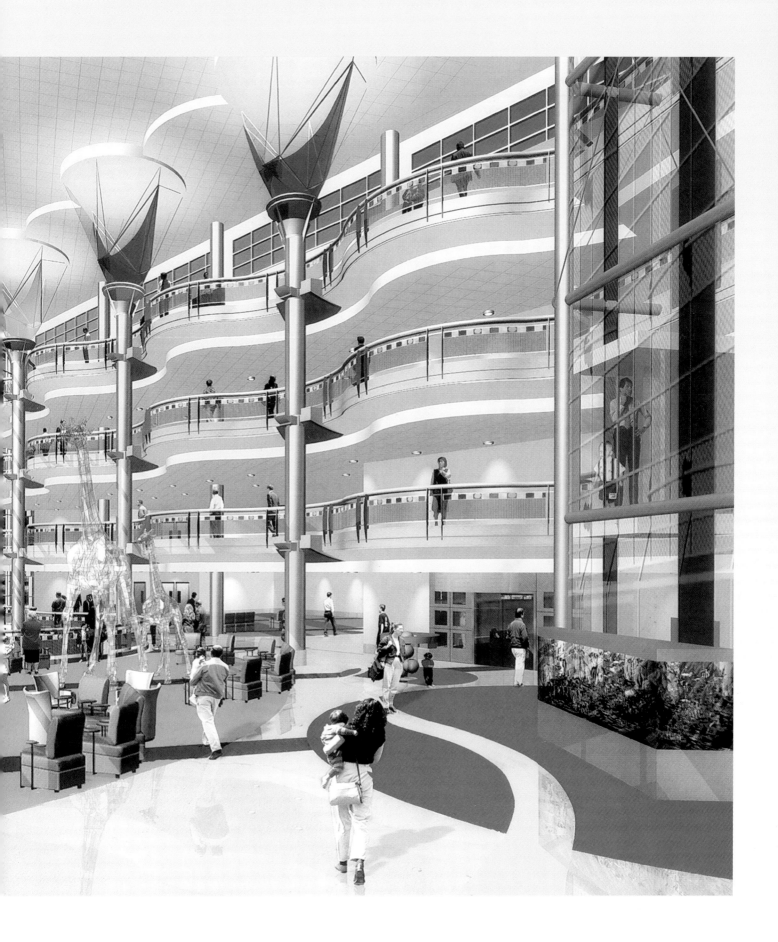

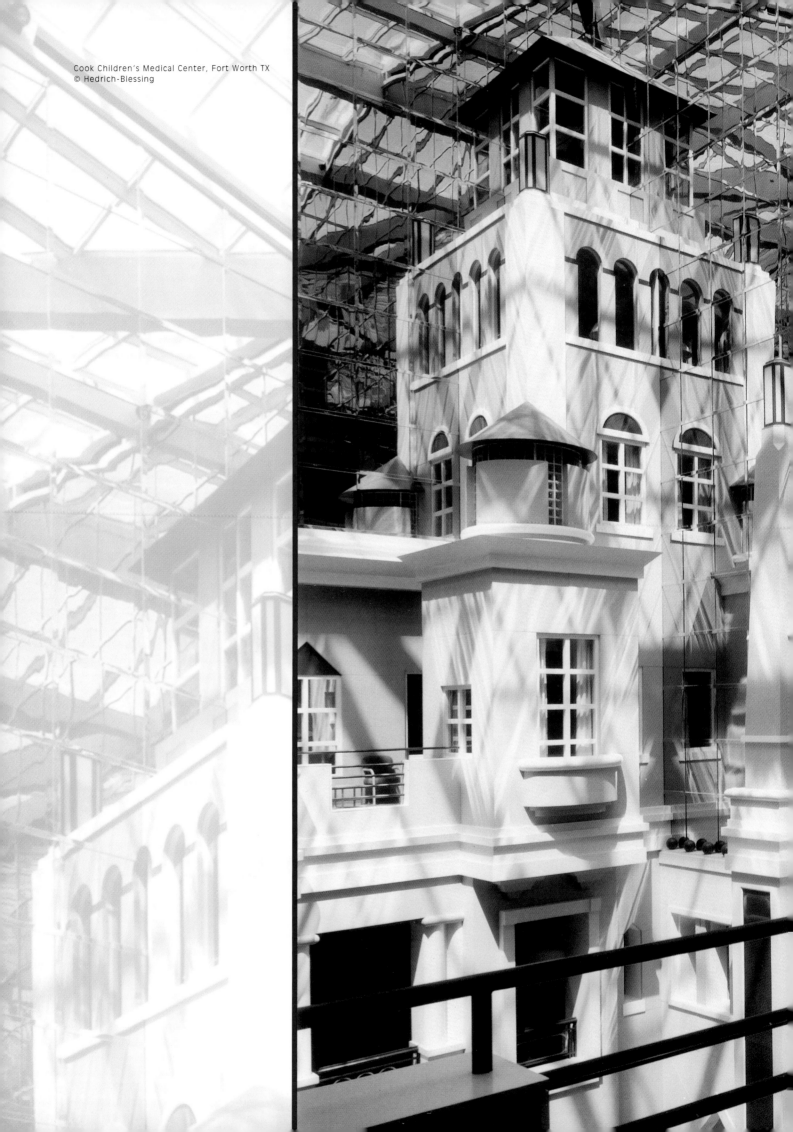

Cook Children's Medical Center, Fort Worth TX
© Hedrich-Blessing

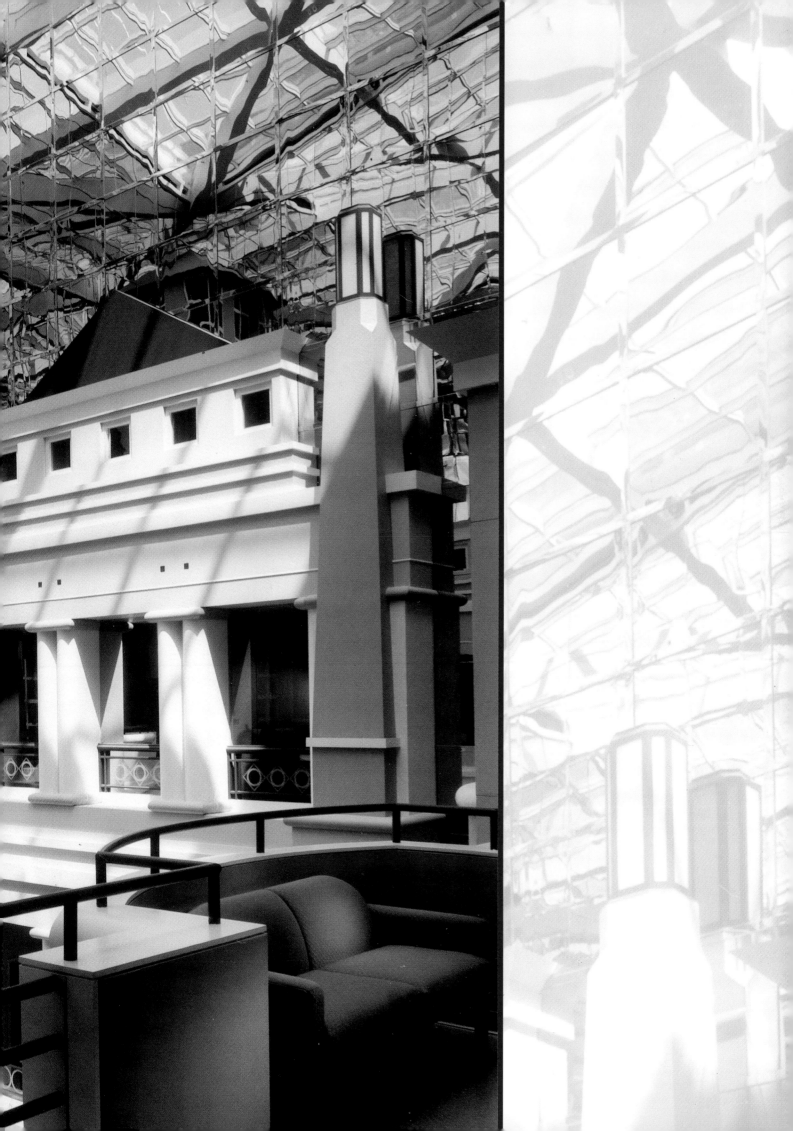

Atrium, major expansion project,
The Hospital for Sick Children,
Toronto, Ontario, Canada
© Lenscape Inc.

72

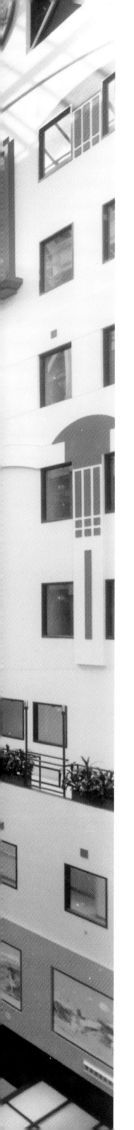

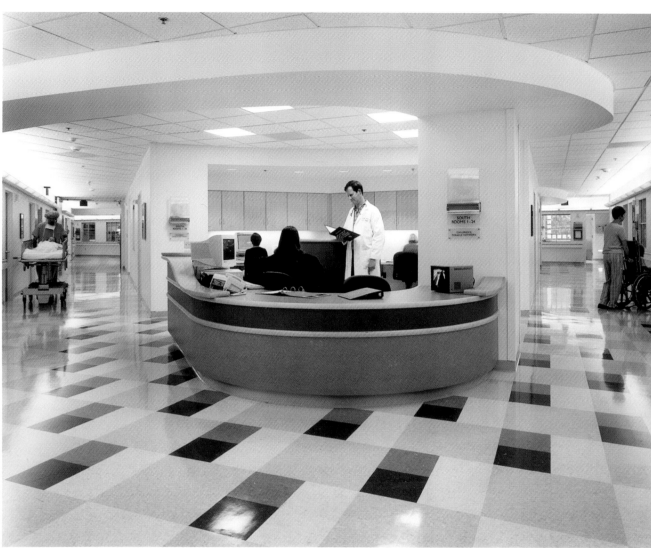

Nurses' station, Doernbecher's Children's Hospital, Portland OR © Eckert & Eckert

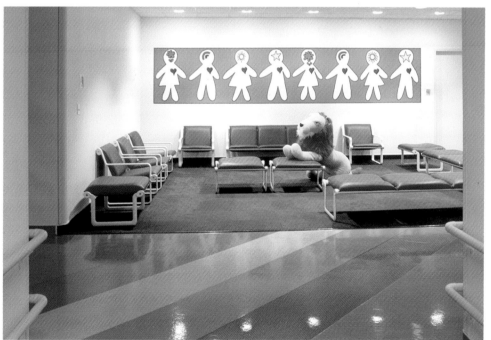

Waiting area, Texas Scottish Rite Hospital for Children, Dallas TX
© Roger Bell

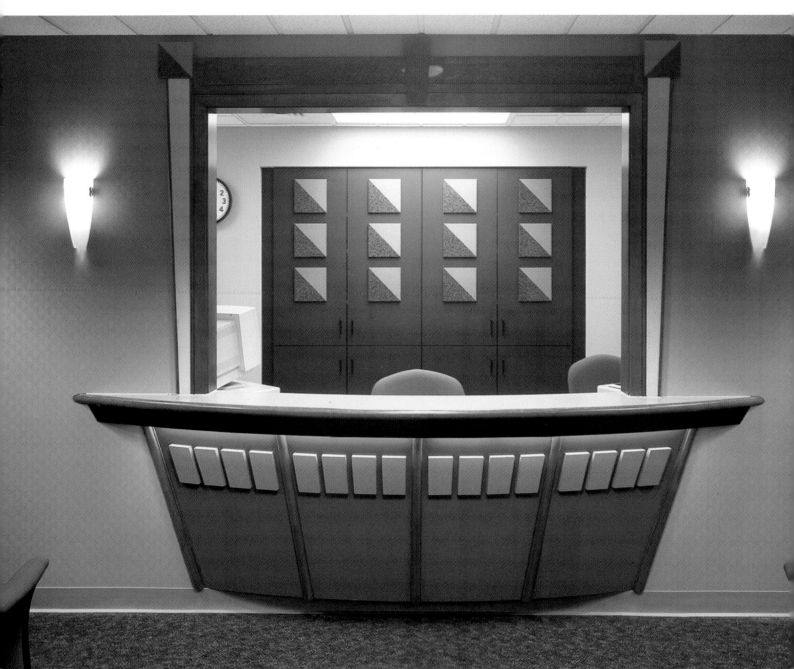

Reception/Nurses' station, Vanderbilt Children's Hospital, Nashville TN © Bill La Fevor

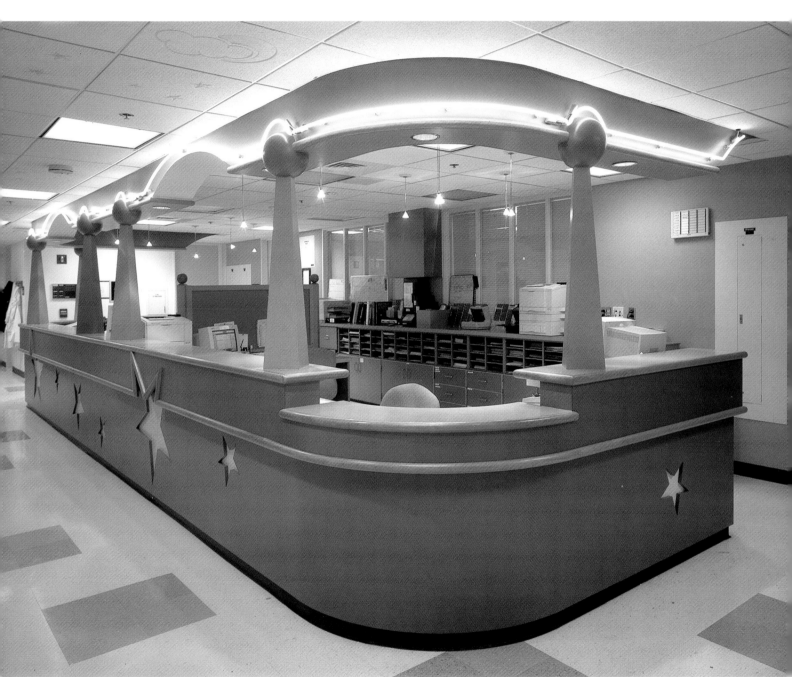

Nurses' station, Vanderbilt Children's Hospital, Nashville TN © Vanderbilt Children's Hospital

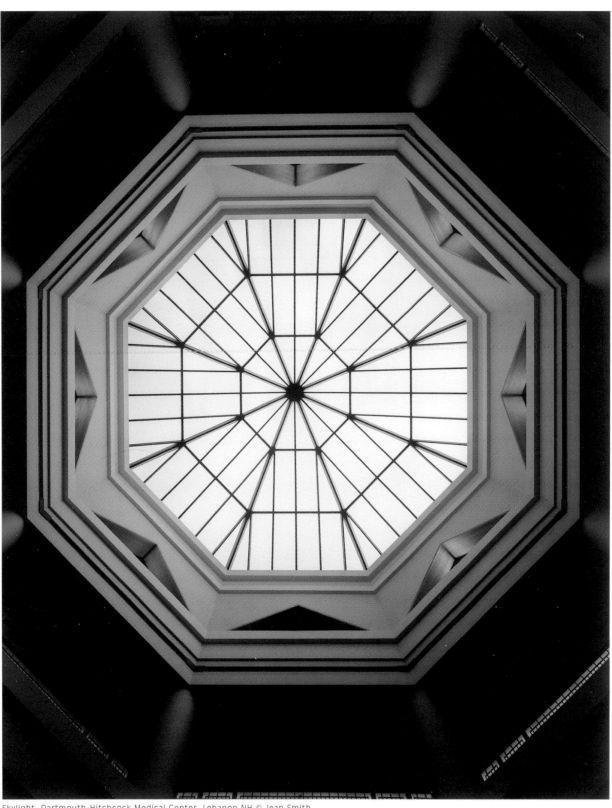

Skylight, Dartmouth-Hitchcock Medical Center, Lebanon NH © Jean Smith

Atrium, major expansion project, Children's Hospital Medical Center of Akron, Akron OH
© Scott McDonald/Hedrich-Blessing

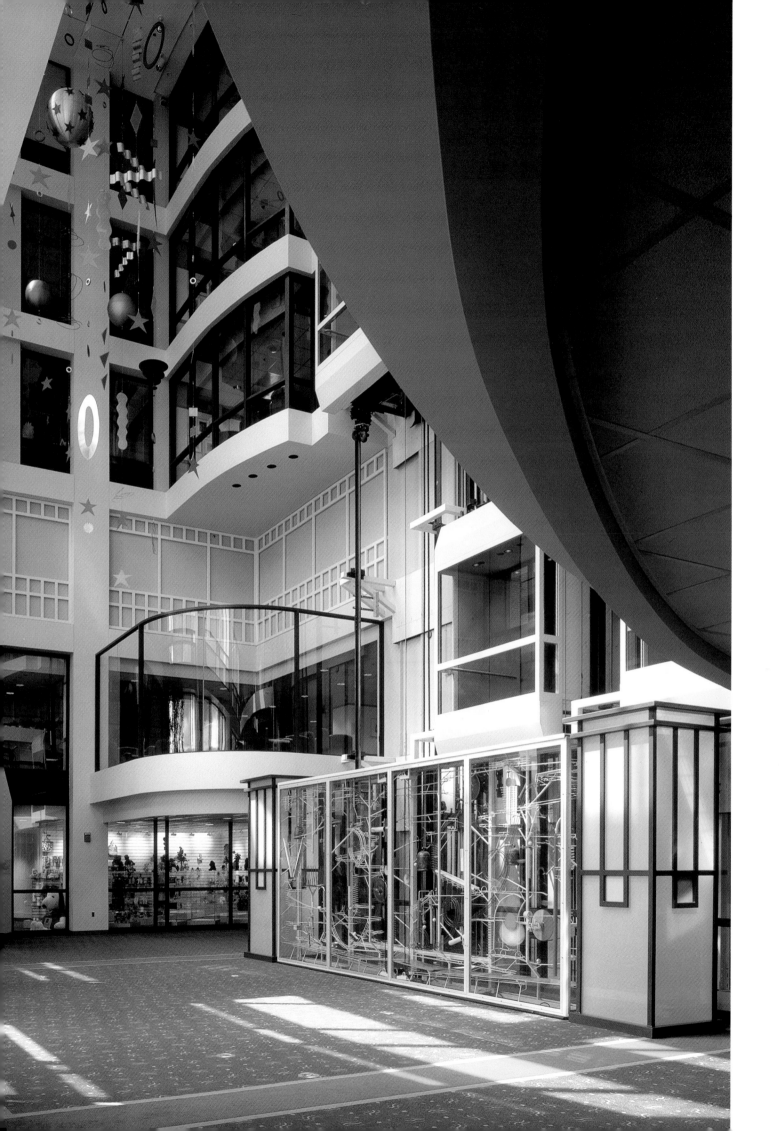

# 3

# Healing
# Environments

The Zoo at
Hasbro Children's
Hospital

A Joint Project Of The Roger Williams Park Zoo,
The Rhode Island Zoological Society,
And Hasbro Children's Hospital.

Therapeutic environments for children must be 'healing environments' —positive, enabling, and compassionate places that enhance their ability to begin the healing process. Children's healthcare providers should be advocates for children and their families and be committed to providing them with the highest standards of family-centered care. In order to achieve this level of care, healing partnerships must exist between patients and caregivers, patients and families, and patients and the care environment.

Environments are never neutral. In the healthcare setting, it is imperative that the facility is designed to assist children with handling the stress and emotions associated with illness. The enlightened healthcare provider not only accommodates the patient's basic medical needs, but also the physical, social, psychological, and developmental needs of children.

Designers of therapeutic environments for children must be aware of the influence their design will have on the healing process. While there is no formula for a 'healing environment,' looking across the behavior sciences and health fields, several factors are substantiated to be effective in promoting wellness. Healing environments that promote health and wellness encourage an integration of mind, body, and spirit by providing appropriate opportunities for privacy, dignity, self-esteem, identity, social support, and security. This can be achieved by designing environments that foster the following:

- Opportunities for movement—permit children to freely locate spaces, assume different postures, create boundaries, reach new territories, and manifest power;

- Comfort, security and stimulation—create variety and change in the child's sensory environment;

- Control and identity—allow the children some ownership of their environment by controlling visual, acoustic, and lighting levels;

- Access to the child's social support network—provide comfortable accommodation for his/her family members and caregivers; and,

- Positive distractions—incorporate elements that elicit uplifting emotions without stressing the child. The most successful distractions include music, art, laughter, nature scenes, and visits from pets and other non-threatening animals.

To date, the potential of the environment to enhance therapeutic goals has been grossly under-emphasized. Research continues to provide evidence that there is a strong correlation between stress and illness and that a positive attitude can facilitate the healing process. Consequently, as much devotion should be given to the quality of the environment imposed on children during their hospital stay as is given to their medical care.

John Pangrazio, FAIA
NBBJ
Seattle WA

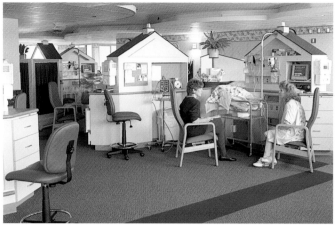

Above and below: NICU Children's Medical Center, Dayton OH
© Children's Medical Center

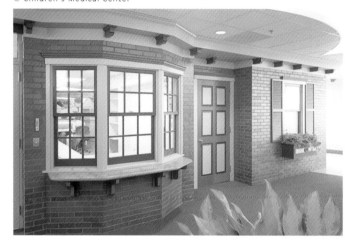

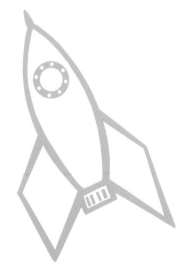

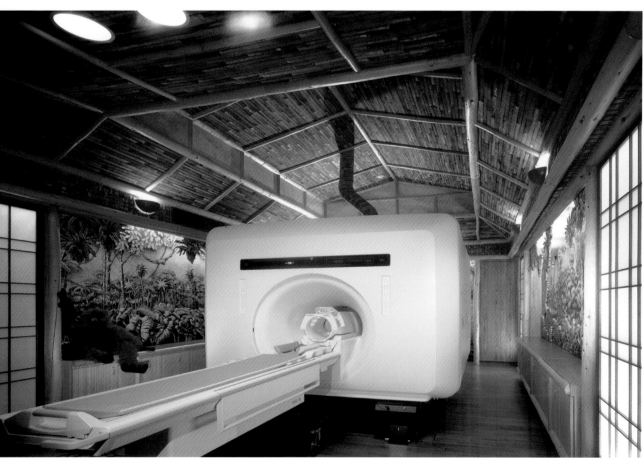

Above and opposite: MRI Jungle, Children's Hospital and Health Center, San Diego CA
© Children's Hospital and Health Center

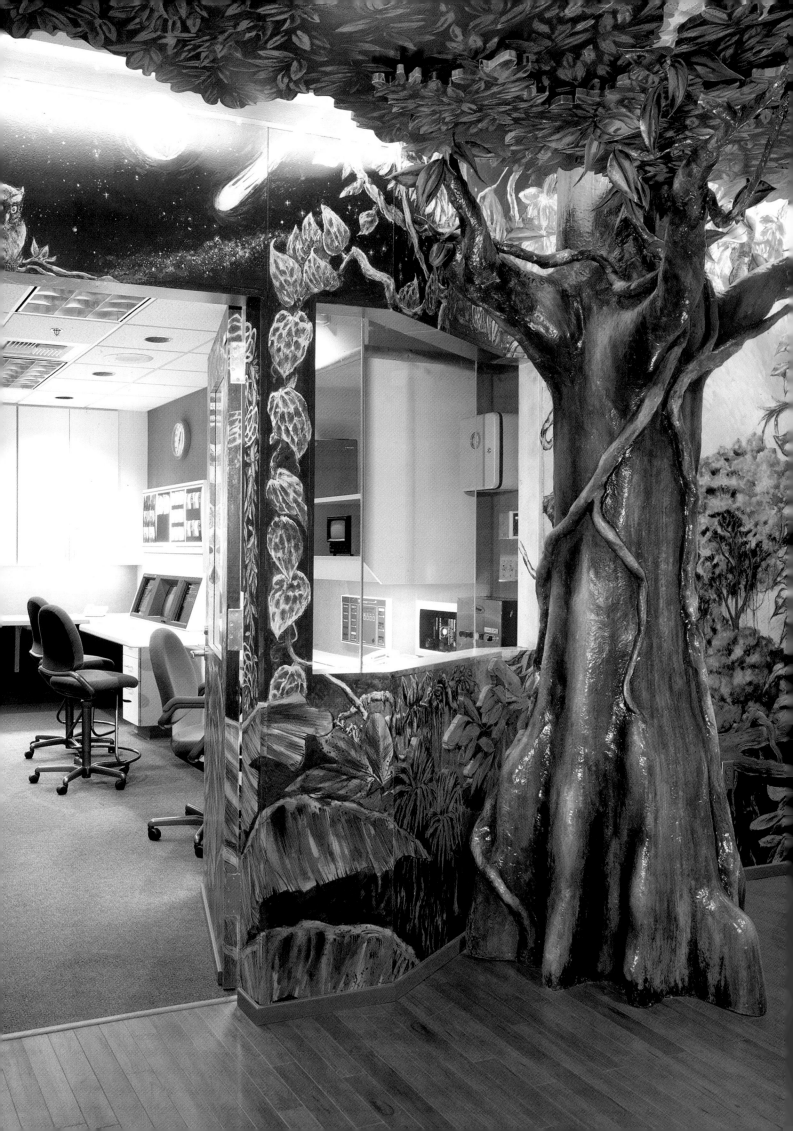

MRI Jungle, Children's Hospital and
Health Center, San Diego CA
© Children's Hospital and Health Center

82

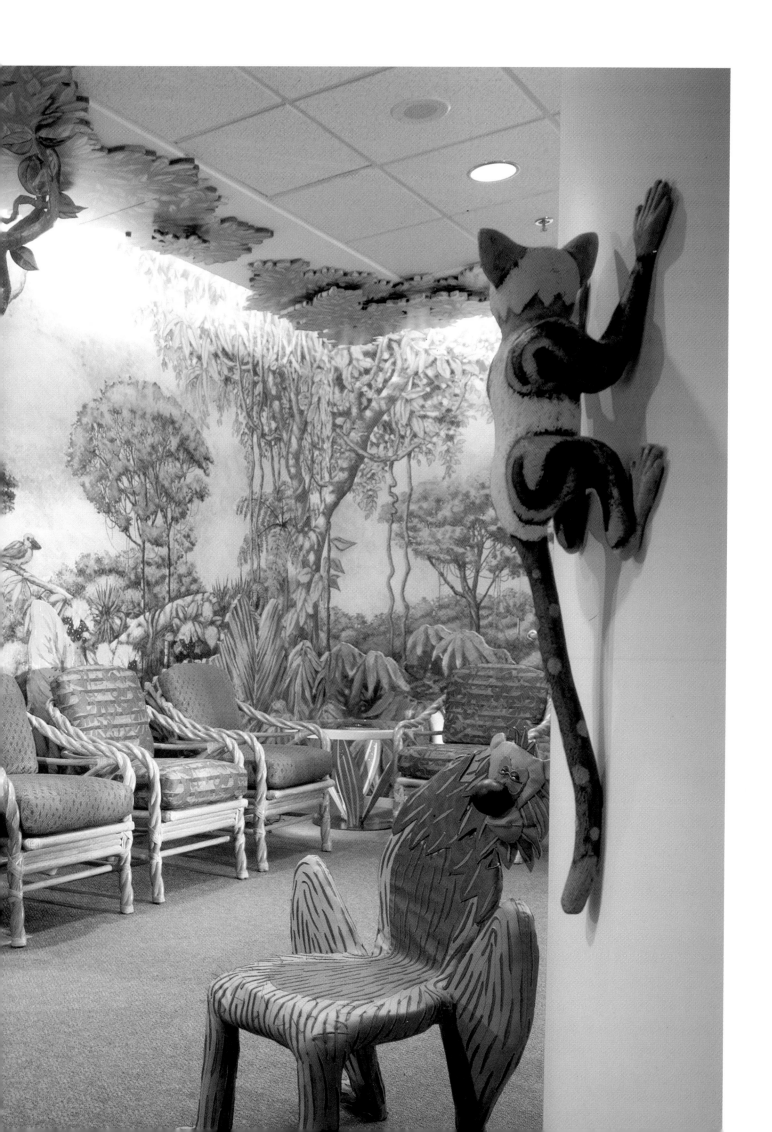

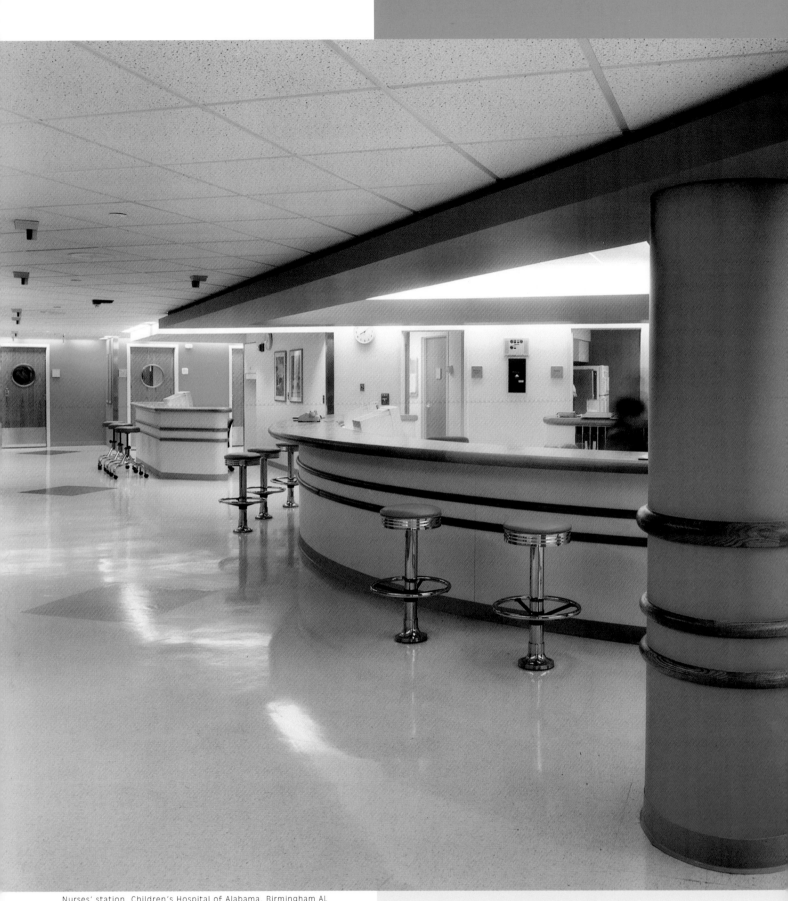

Nurses' station, Children's Hospital of Alabama, Birmingham AL
© Children's Hospital of Alabama

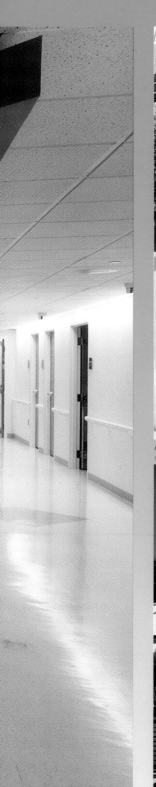

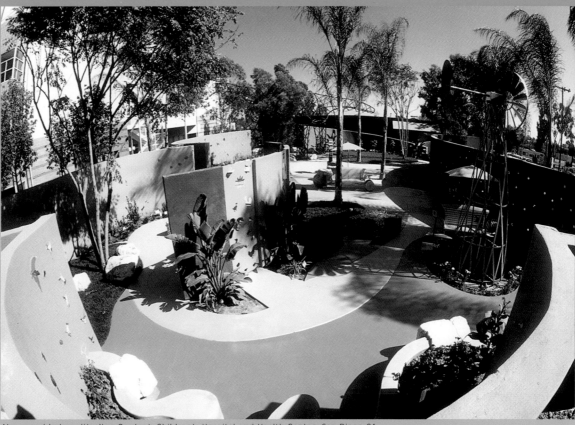

Above and below: 'Healing Garden', Children's Hospital and Health Center, San Diego CA
© Children's Hospital and Health Center

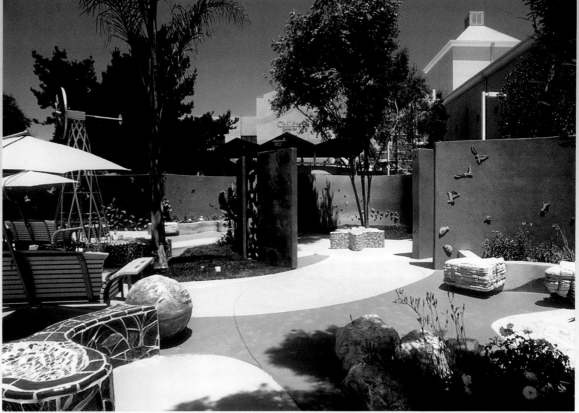

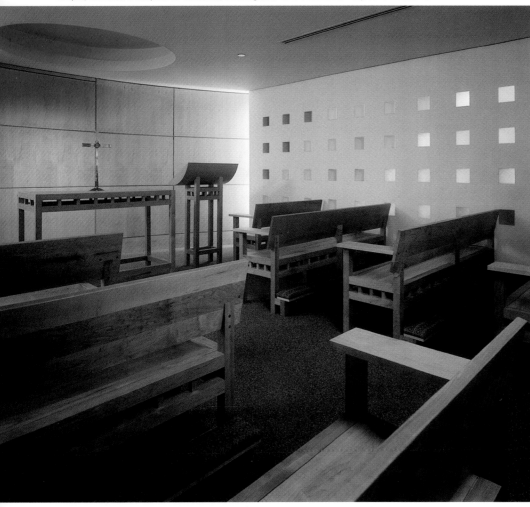

The real 'Patch Adams M.D.' provides advice on humour in healthcare, Westchester Medical Center
© Westchester Medical Center

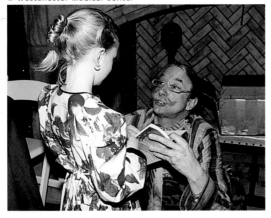

Chapel, Le Bonheur Children's Medical Center, Memphis TN
© Le Bonheur Children's Medical Center

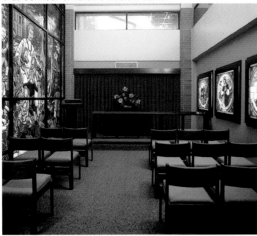

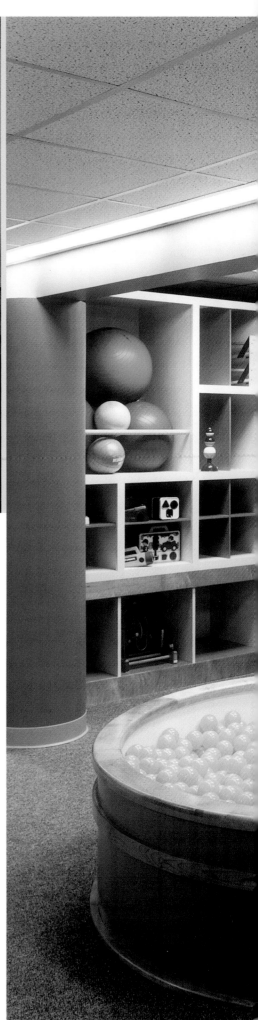

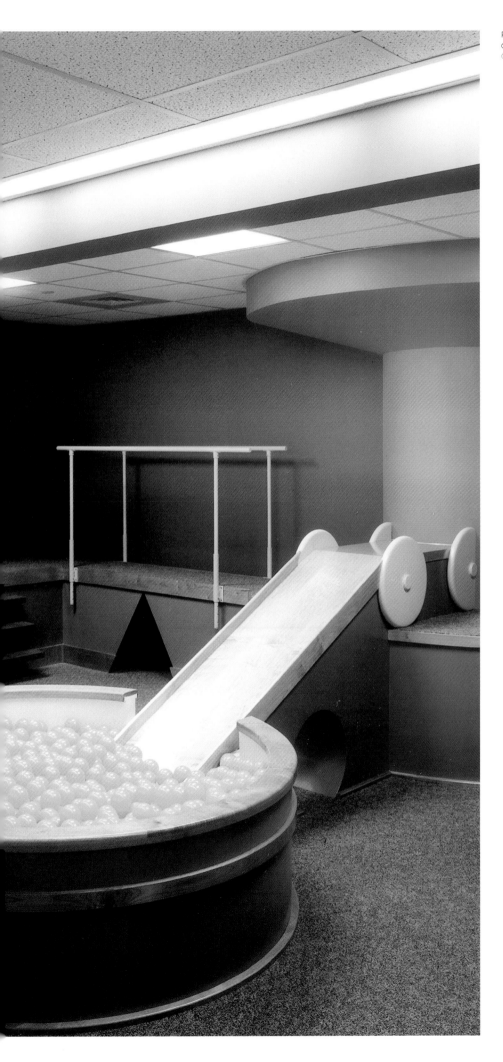

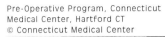

Pre-Operative Program, Connecticut
Medical Center, Hartford CT
© Connecticut Medical Center

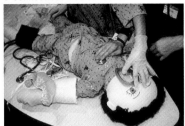

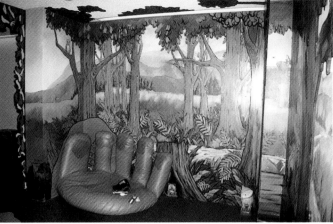

'Glove Chair', San Diego Children's Hospital, San Diego CA
© San Diego Children's Hospital

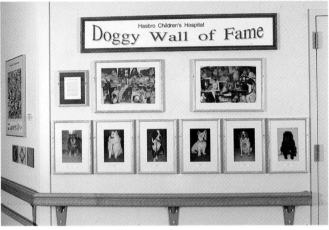

Doggy Wall of Fame, Hasbro Children's Hospital, Providence RI
© Lou Trombetti

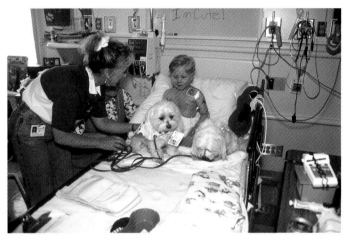

Pet Therapy Program, Children's Hospital and Health Center, San Diego CA
© Children's Hospital and Health Center

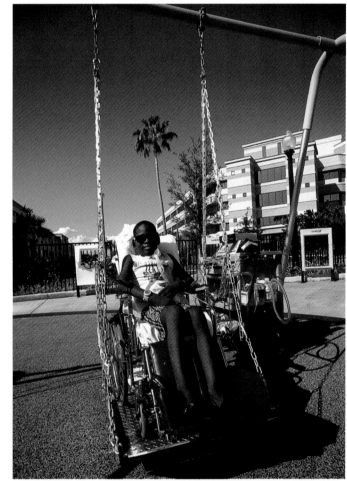

Following pages:
The World's first in-hospital zoo,
Hasbro Children's Hospital, Providence RI
© Lou Trombetti

'Swing for all,' All Children's Hospital, St Petersburgh FL
© All Children's Hospital

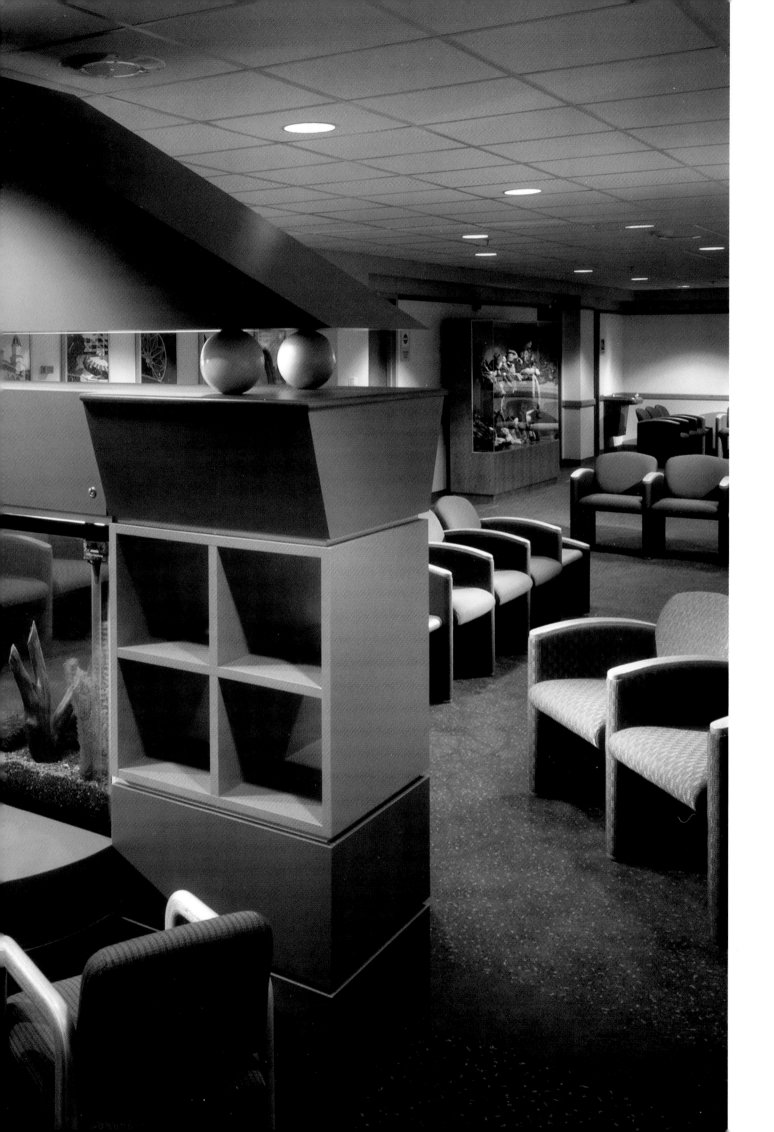

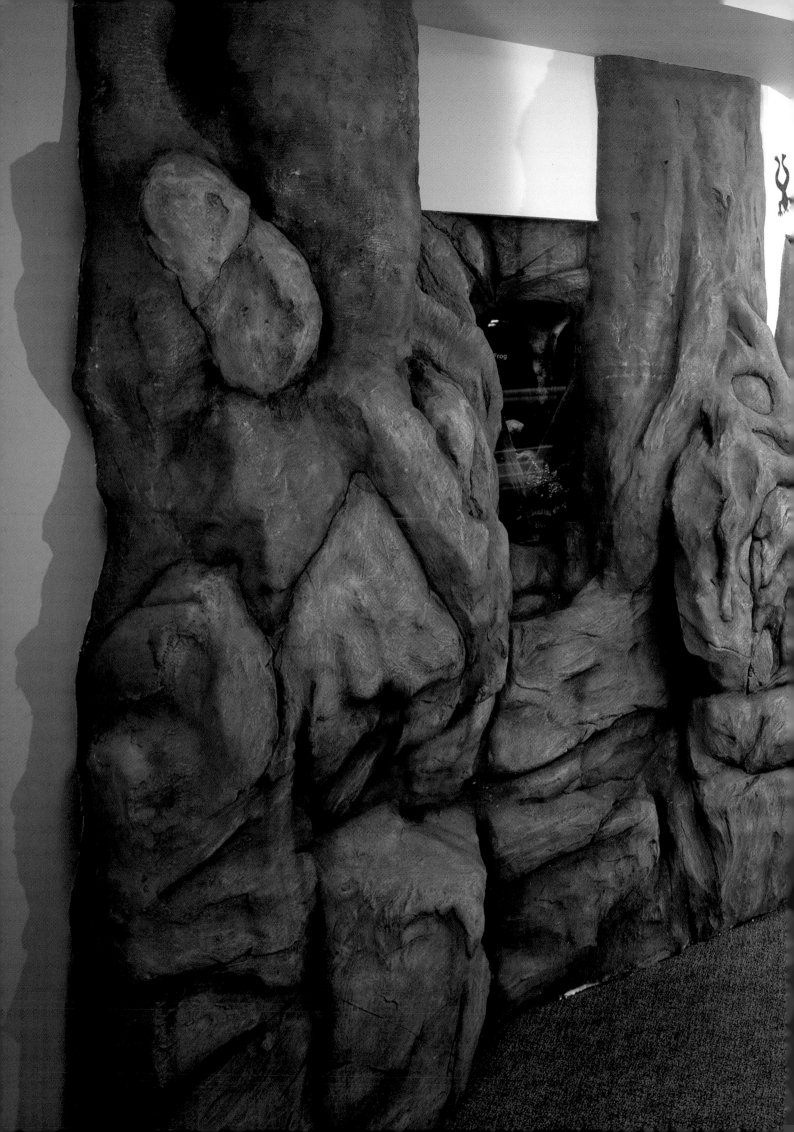

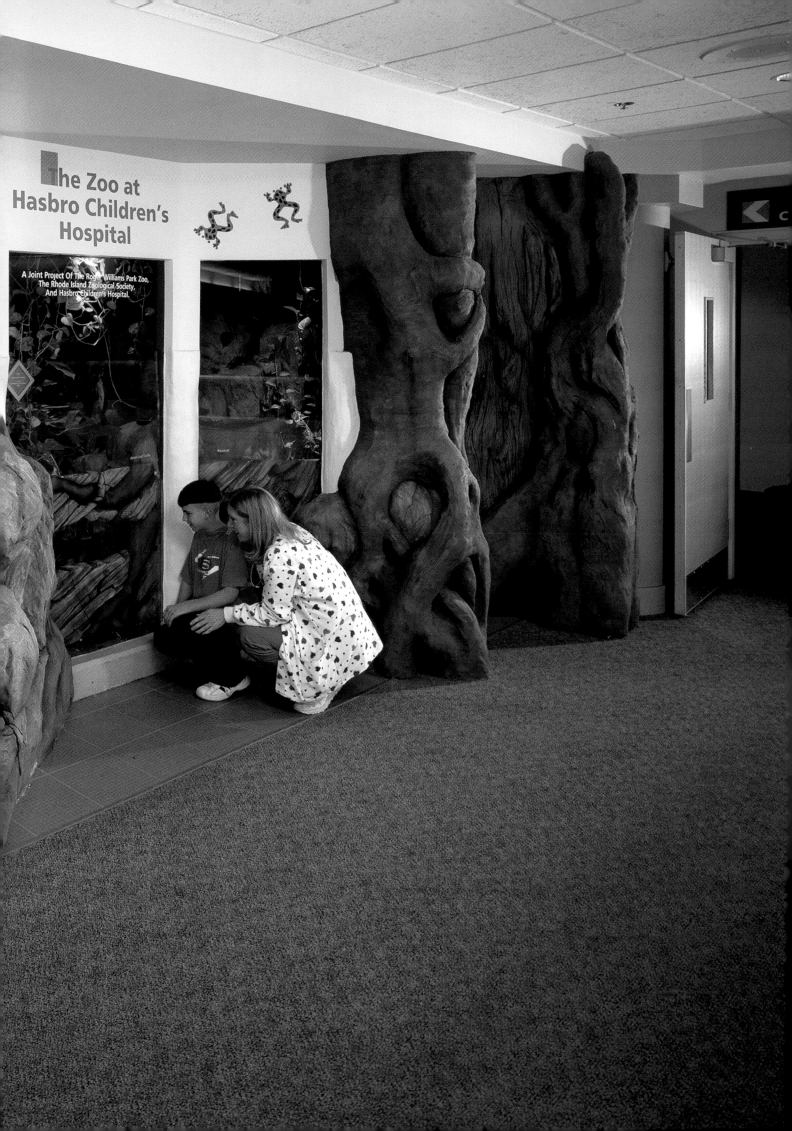

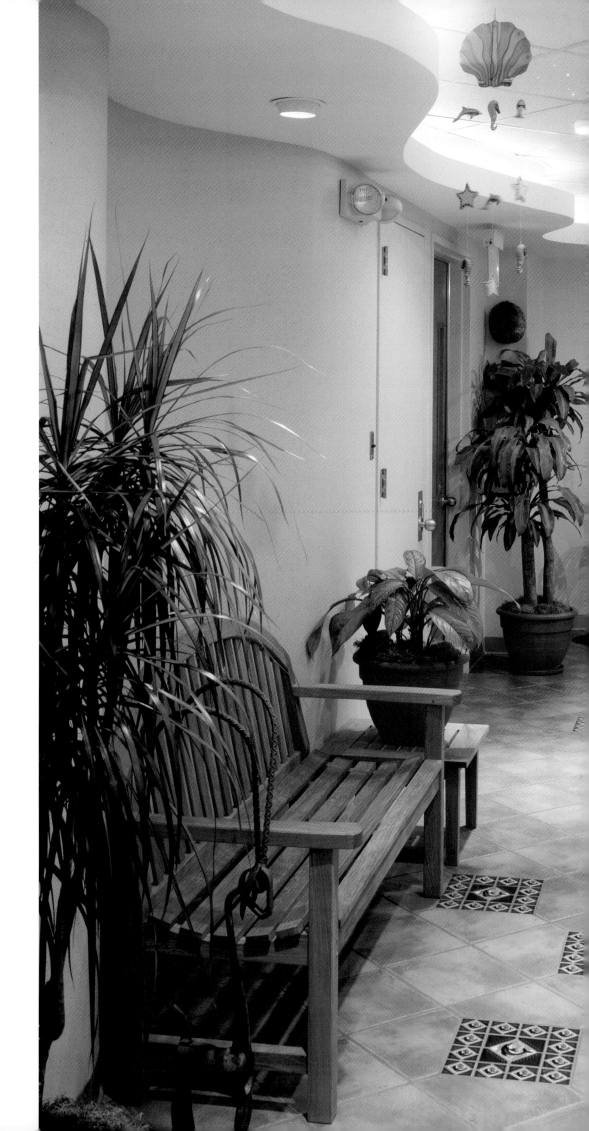

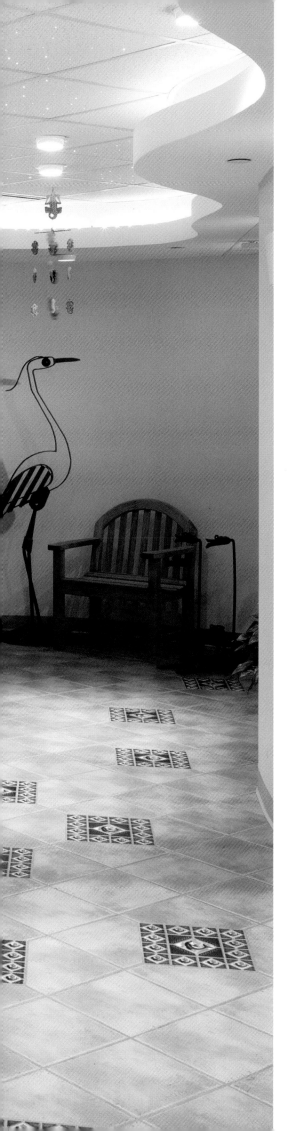

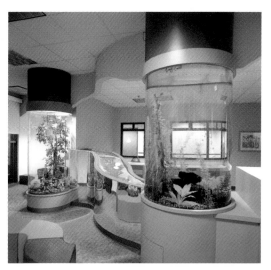

Fish tank in waiting area,
Valley Children's Hospital, Madera CA
© Kelly Peterson

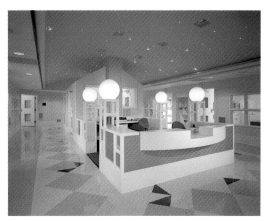

Nurses' station,
Children's Hospital and Health
Center, San Diego CA
© Children's Hospital
and Health Center

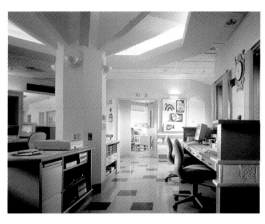

Nurses' station,
Hasbro Children's Hospital,
Providence RI
© Robert Miller

Waiting area, St Louis Children's Hospital, St Louis MO
© William E Mathis

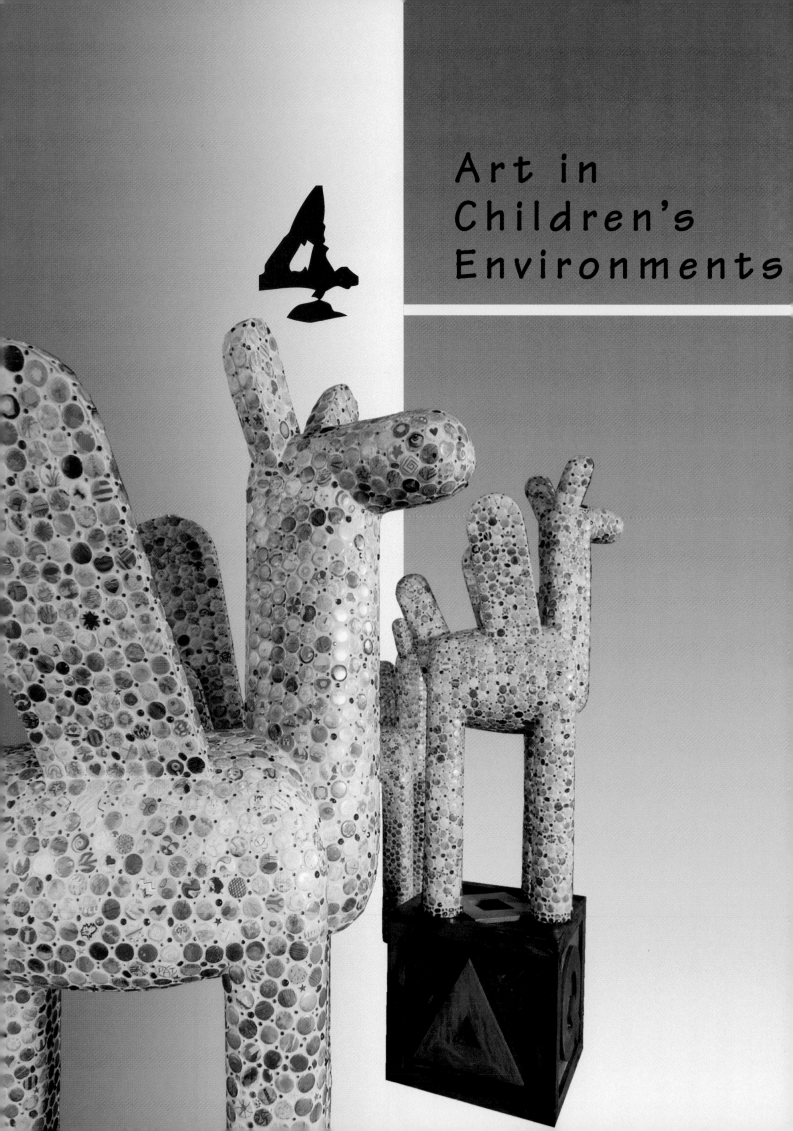

# 4

# Art in Children's Environments

Artwork, like any component of the design process, should be tied to the design vocabulary of the entire healthcare facility. Its overall role in the design solution should relate to the function and the institution's delivery of care philosophy. If an interactive art element is installed and the commitment to maintaining or keeping it operational is lacking, then it does more harm than good.

Building a children's hospital should not be about building a structure, but about building a place where children's health concerns are recognized, addressed, and accommodated. It should be known in the community as a trusted resource, a brand that promises to protect, heal and keep well, its most valuable resource. Whether it is a trauma or an elective procedure that causes a patient to enter the health system, the path to care must be clear, calming, and considerate of not only patients, but of their family and caregivers as well.

Environments for children should be less about animation and more about the needs of a special population. Details should be safe and maintainable. They should provide interest and education, but not over stimulation. They should always involve the family or caregiver.

A successful approach is to link an art program to the community it serves. Volunteers at the Children's Hospital at Yale New Haven in New Haven, Connecticut went to art schools around the world and asked for donations of art that depicted a 'Tale of Courage.' Twenty-six hundred pieces, many in groupings, were donated. A private donor paid for the framing of the entire collection. The collection is priceless. Another example is Hasbro Children's Hospital in Providence, Rhode Island, where a collection was also created from a community. An artist took a sabbatical from his teaching position to attempt to have children in every elementary school in Rhode Island create a 6" x 6" ceramic tile. The 11,000 tiles created were built into the walls of corridors and nurse stations, creating a 'Circle of Clay' that will tie these families and the community to the hospital for generations to come.

All children's hospitals should be seen as a resource center for wellness, good health and family care. From a child's eyes, it should be a facility for healthy development; for parents it should be for family growth; for the community, it should be a valuable resource to nurture and share. Artwork is needed to achieve that goal.

**Rosalyn Cama, FASID**
President ASID
Washington D.C.

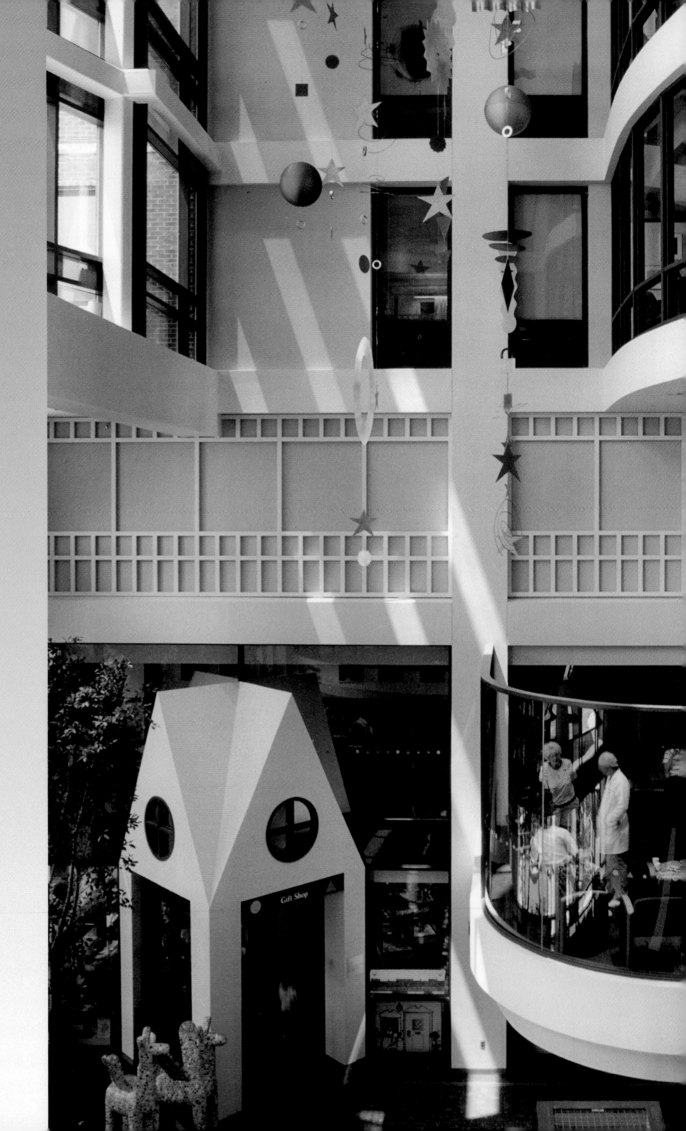

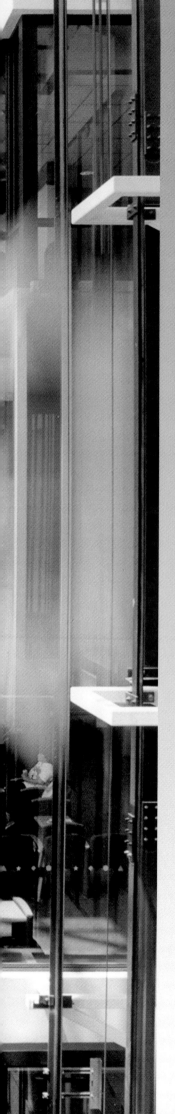

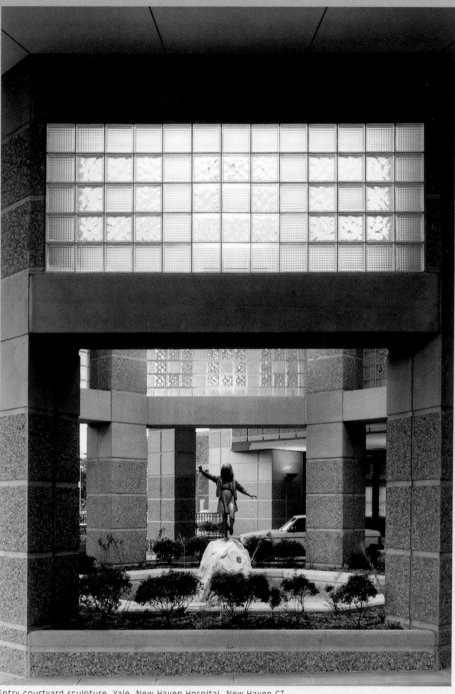

Entry courtyard sculpture, Yale, New Haven Hospital, New Haven CT
© Peter Aaron/Esto Photographics

Atrium, Children's Hospital Medical Center, Akron OH © Feinknopf

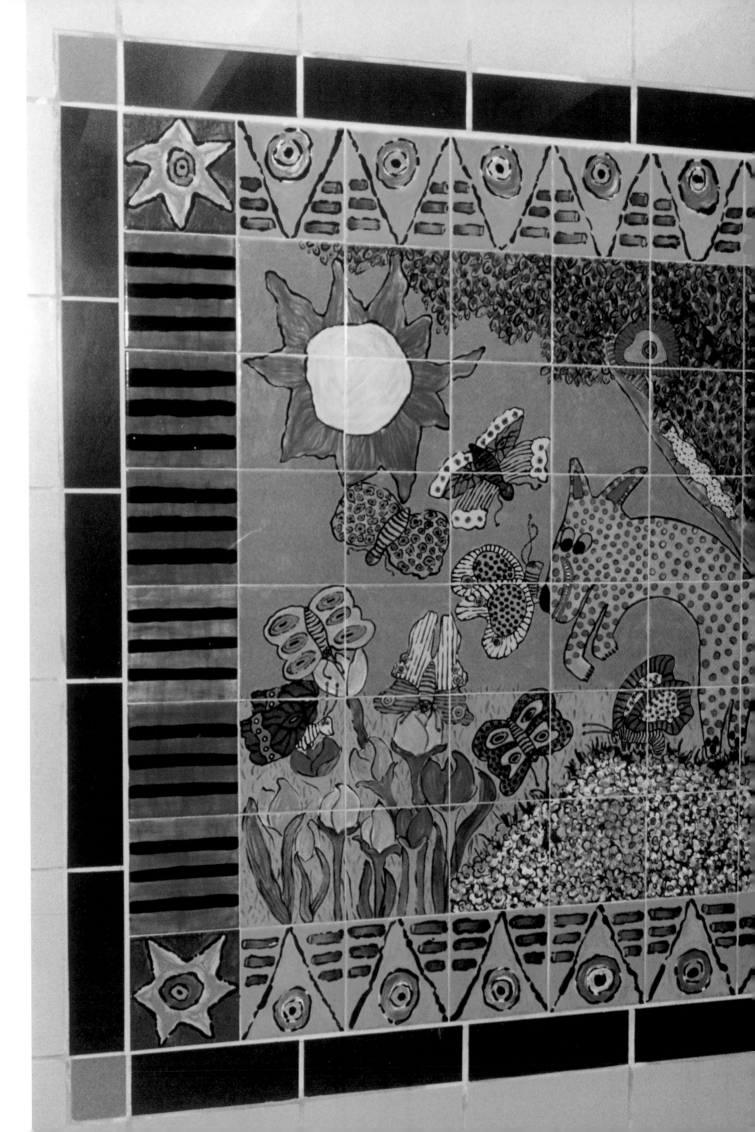

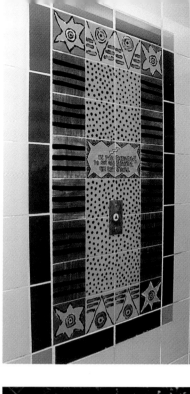

Opposite and left: Tile by elevator,
Le Bonheur Children's Medical Center, Memphis TN
© Le Bonheur Children's Medical Center

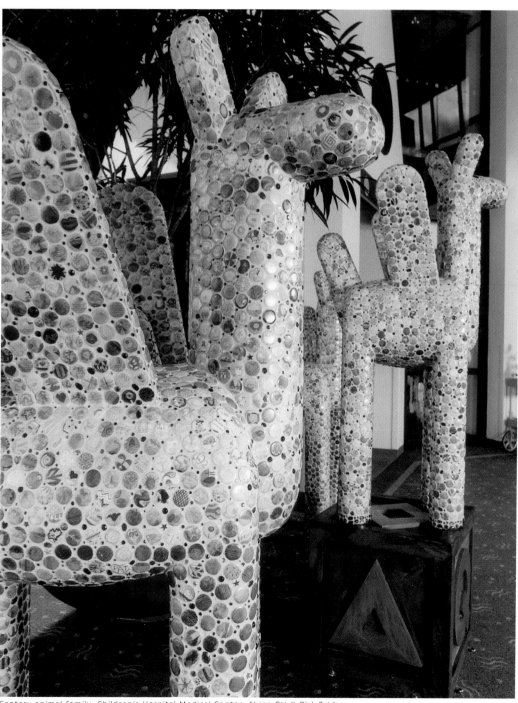

Fantasy animal family, Children's Hospital Medical Center, Akron OH © Rick Zaidan

Tiles, King Triton and the Little Mermaid, Children's Hospital Medical Center, Akron OH © Rick Zaidan

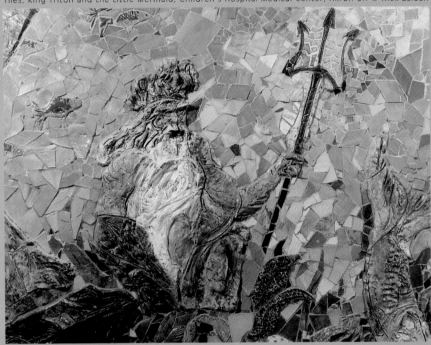

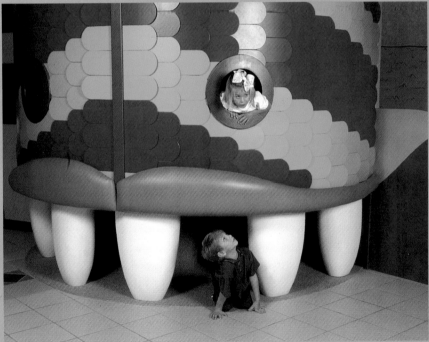

Whale Mural, Le Bonheur Children's Medical Center, Memphis TN © Robert Ames Cook

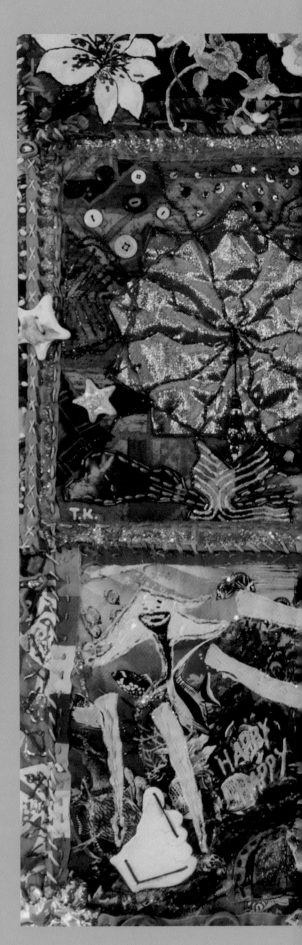

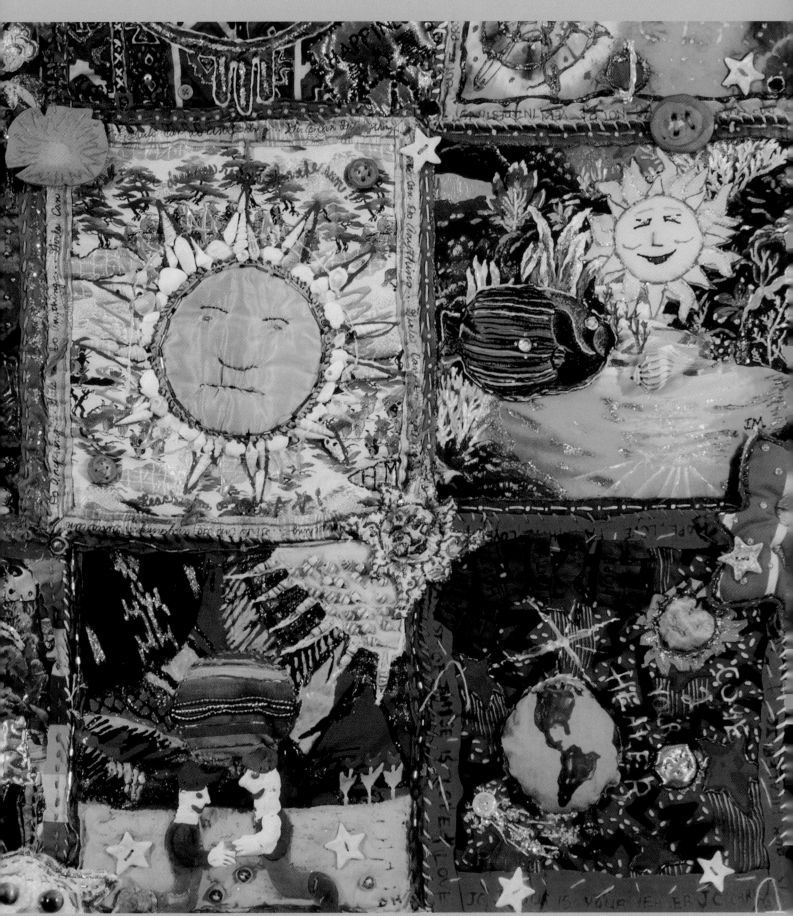

Sunblock 15A Green Quilt, Children's Hospital Medical Center, Akron OH © Rick Zaidan

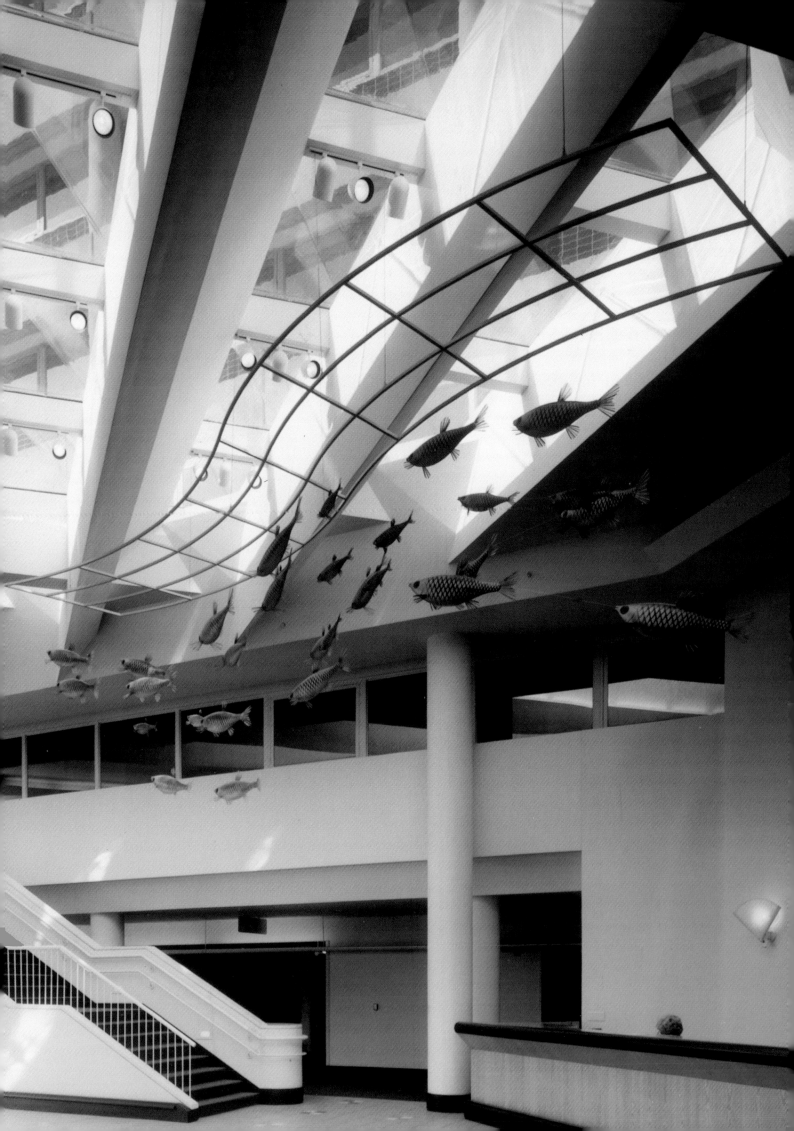

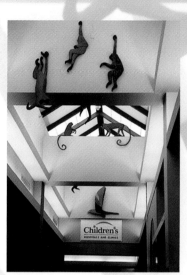

'Monkeys' at entrance to hospital from parking ramp, Children's Hospital and Clinics, Minneapolis MO
© Children's Hospital and Clinics

Fountain, Hasbro Children's Hospital, Providence RI © Jean Smith

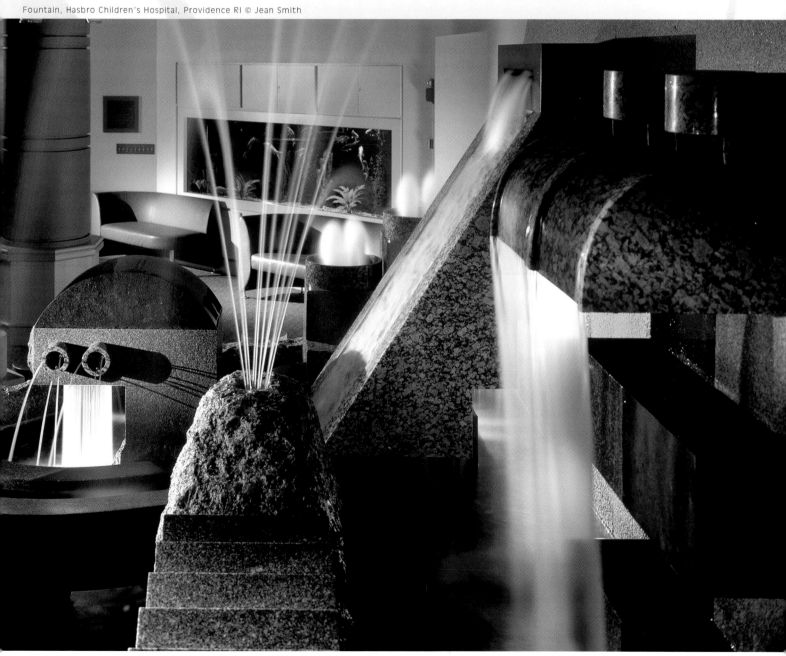

Left: Fish mobile, Children's Hospital of Alabama, Birmingham AL © Children's Hospital of Alabama

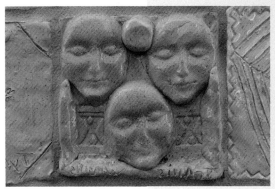

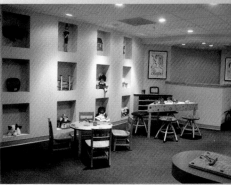

Circle of Clay, Hasbro Children's Hospital, Providence RI
© Lou Trombetti

Waiting area, St Louis Children's Hospital, St Louis MO
© St Louis Children's Hospital

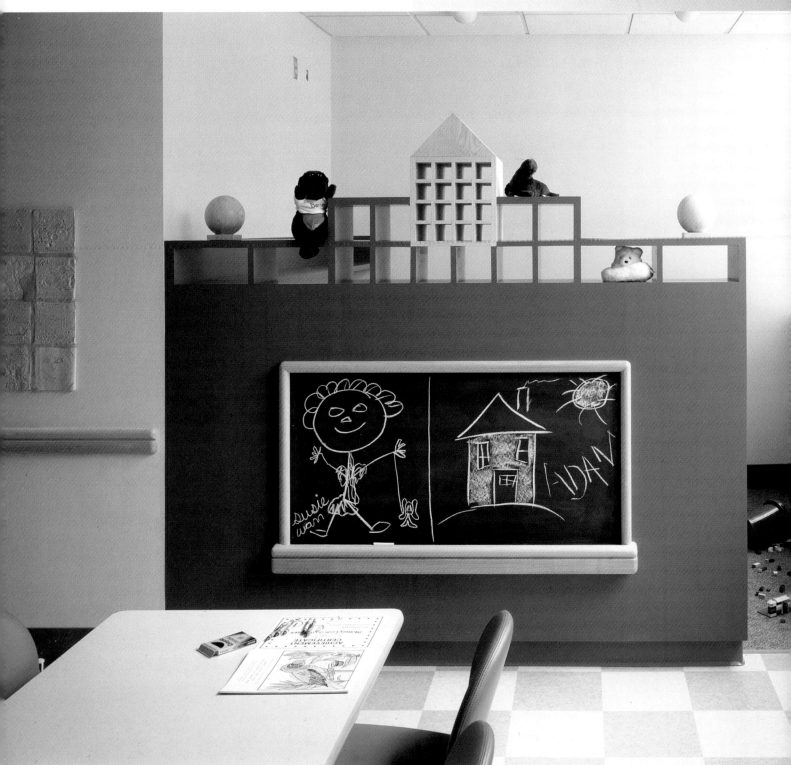

Chemotherapy Clinic chalk board, Hasbro Children's Hospital, Providence RI

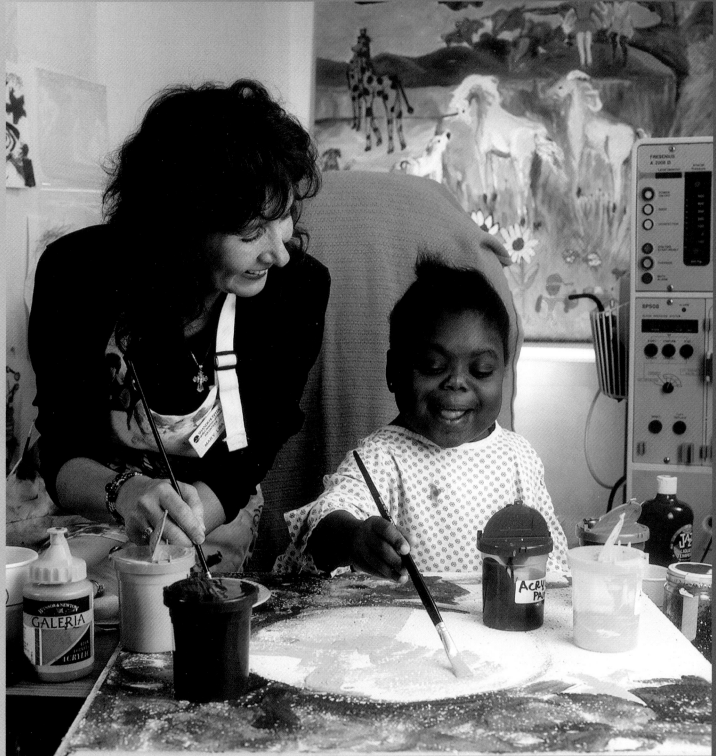

The Art Program, Shands Children's Hospital, Gainesville FL

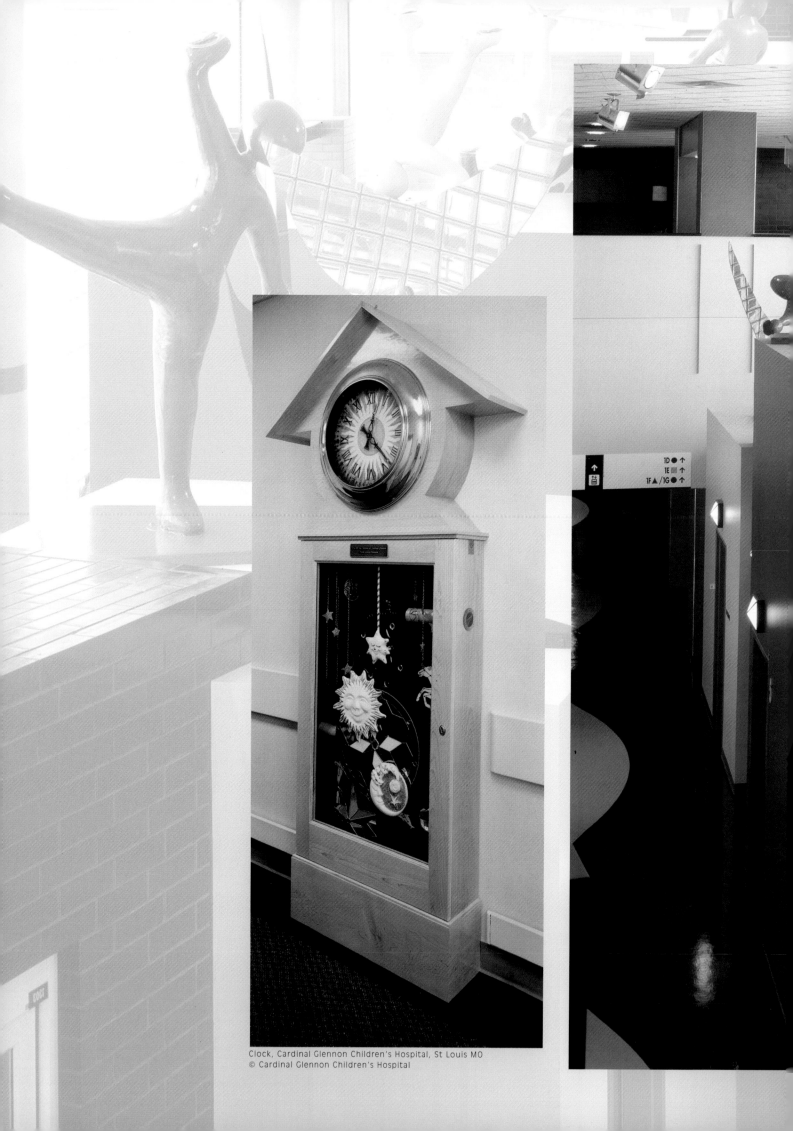

Clock, Cardinal Glennon Children's Hospital, St Louis MO
© Cardinal Glennon Children's Hospital

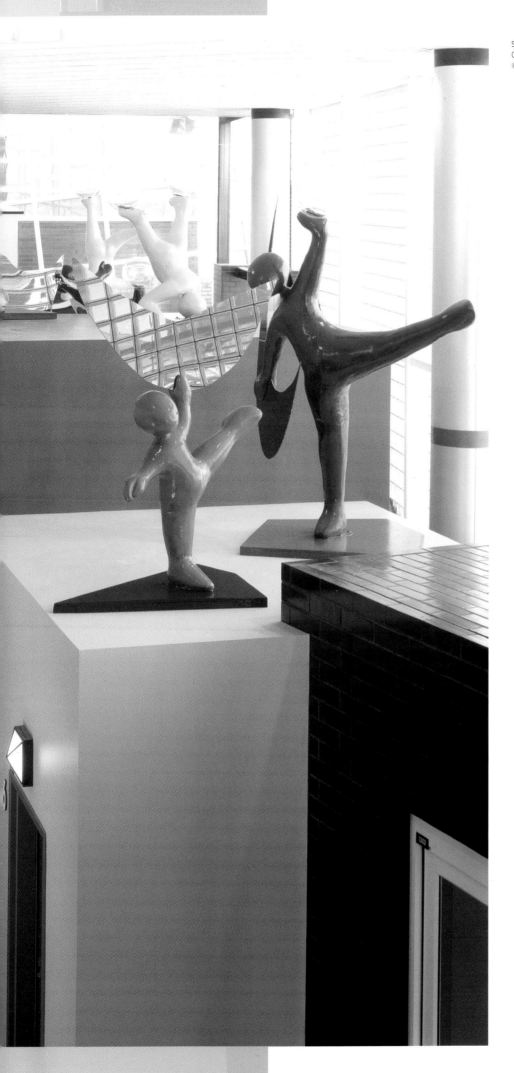

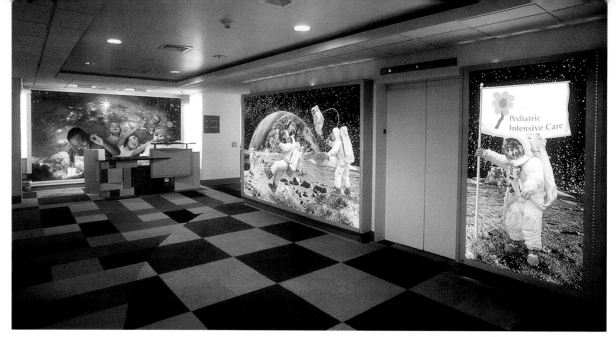

'Clouds', Babies &
Children's Hospital
of New York,
New York NY
© Babies & Children's
Hospital of New York

Digital Photo-mural by Barry Blackman/Tarhill Photo's Inc

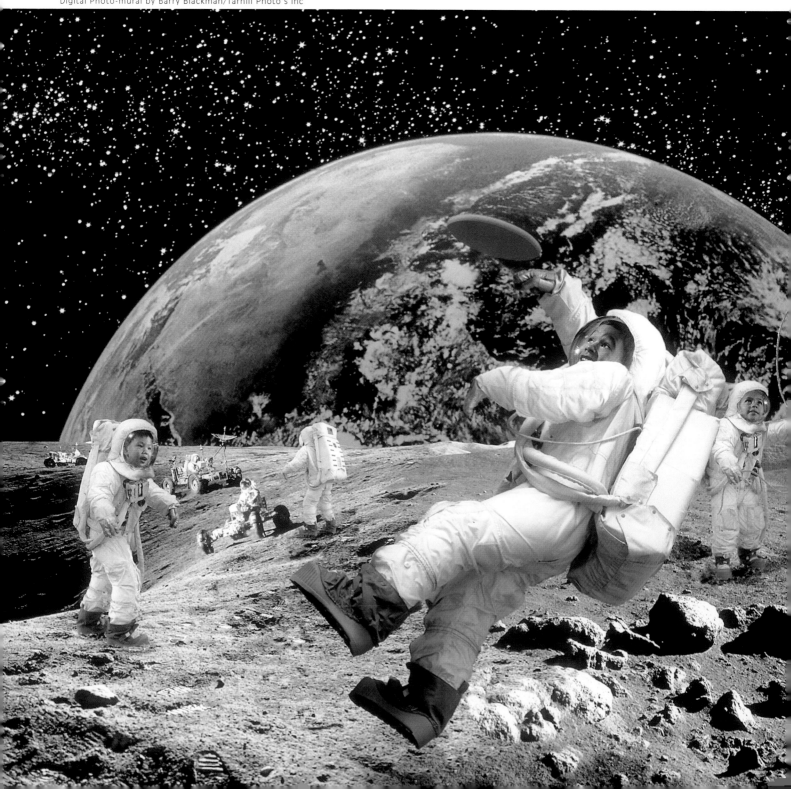

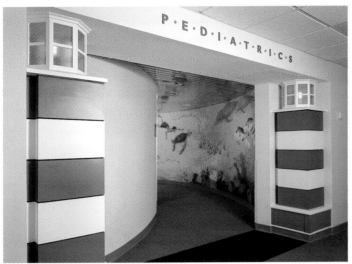

Mural at pediatric entrance by Brooks Pearce, New Hanover Regional Medical Center, Wilmington NC © Jim Stroud

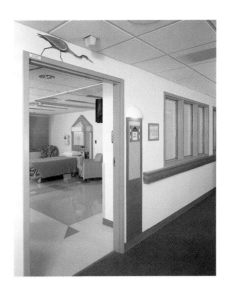

Entrance to room 'bird', New Hanover Regional Medical Center, Wilmington NC © Jim Stroud

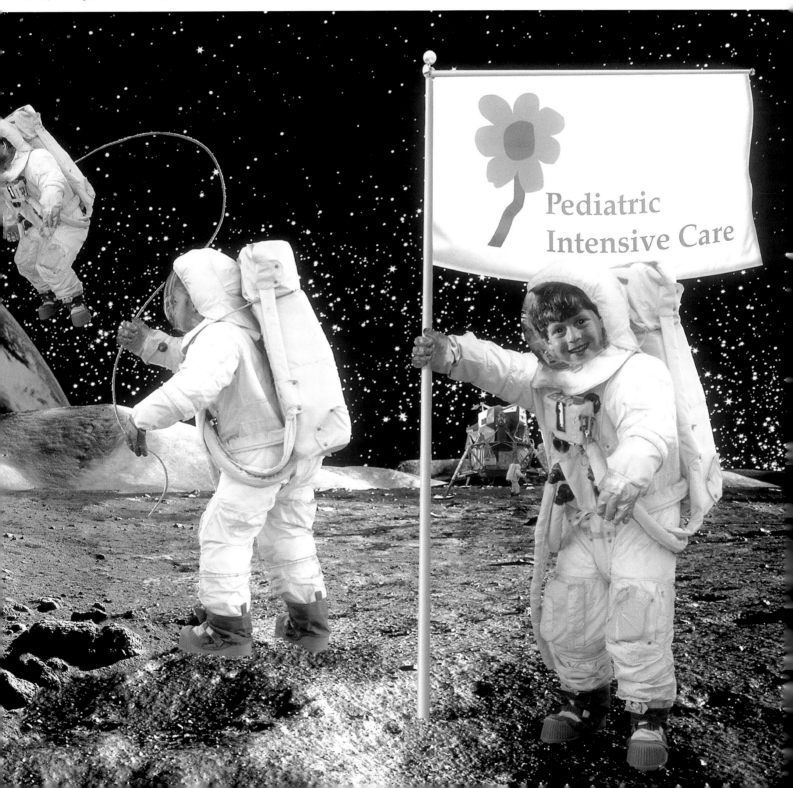

Pediatric Intensive Care

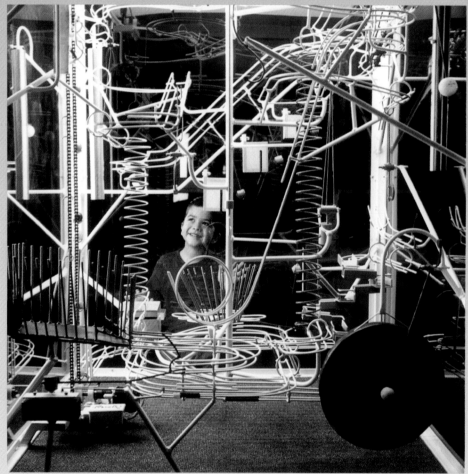

'Incredible Circus', Children's Hospital
and Medical Center, San Diego CA
© Children's Hospital and Medical Center

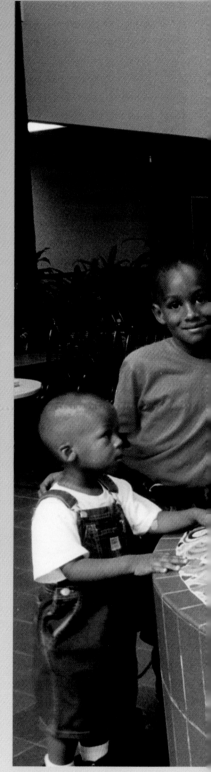

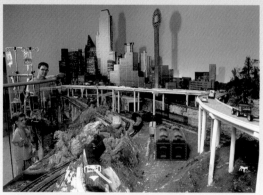

'Trainscape', Children's Medical Center of Dallas, Dallas TX
© Rick Grumbaum

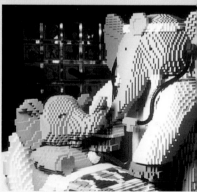

Lego sculpture, Yale, New Haven Hospital,
New Haven CT © Rick Grumbaum

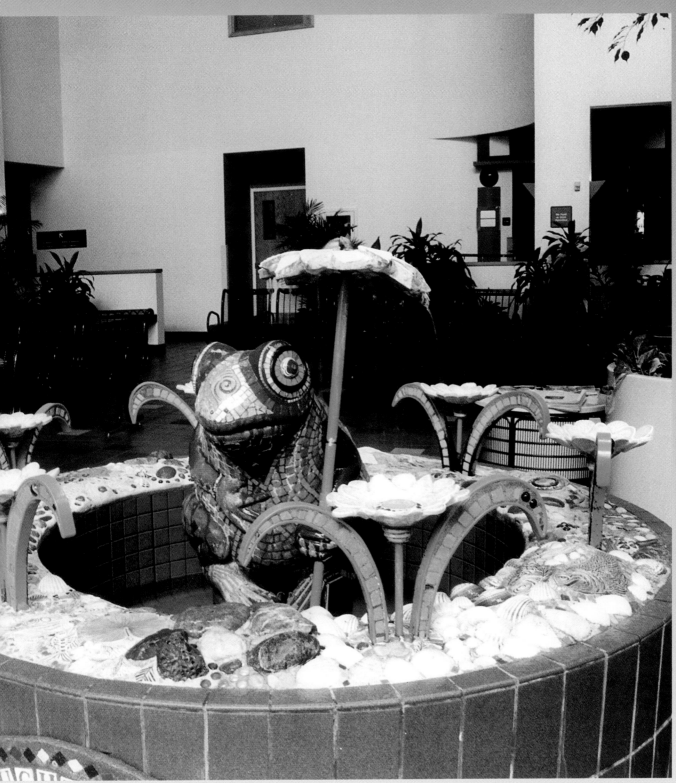

'Frog Fountain', St Christopher's Hospital for Children, Philadelphia PA
© Kimberly Niemela

Following pages: 'Sculpture in motion', Wolfson Children's Hospital, Jacksonville FL
© Wolfson Children's Hospital

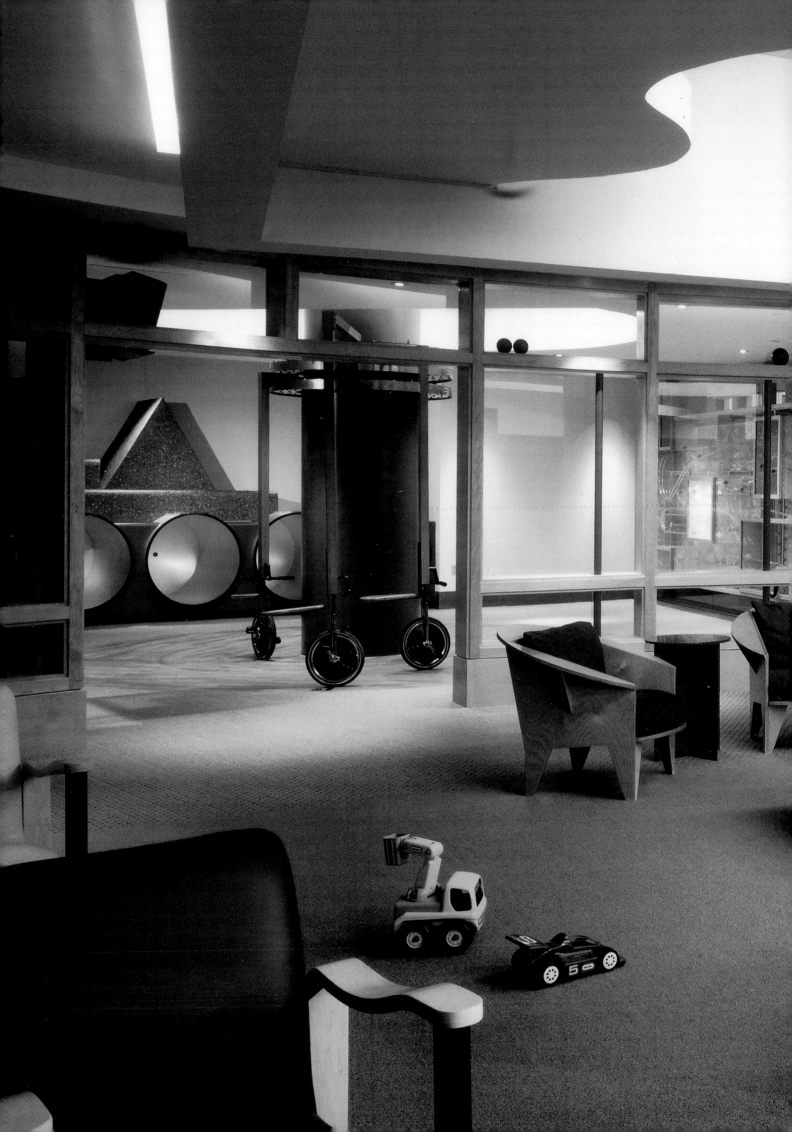

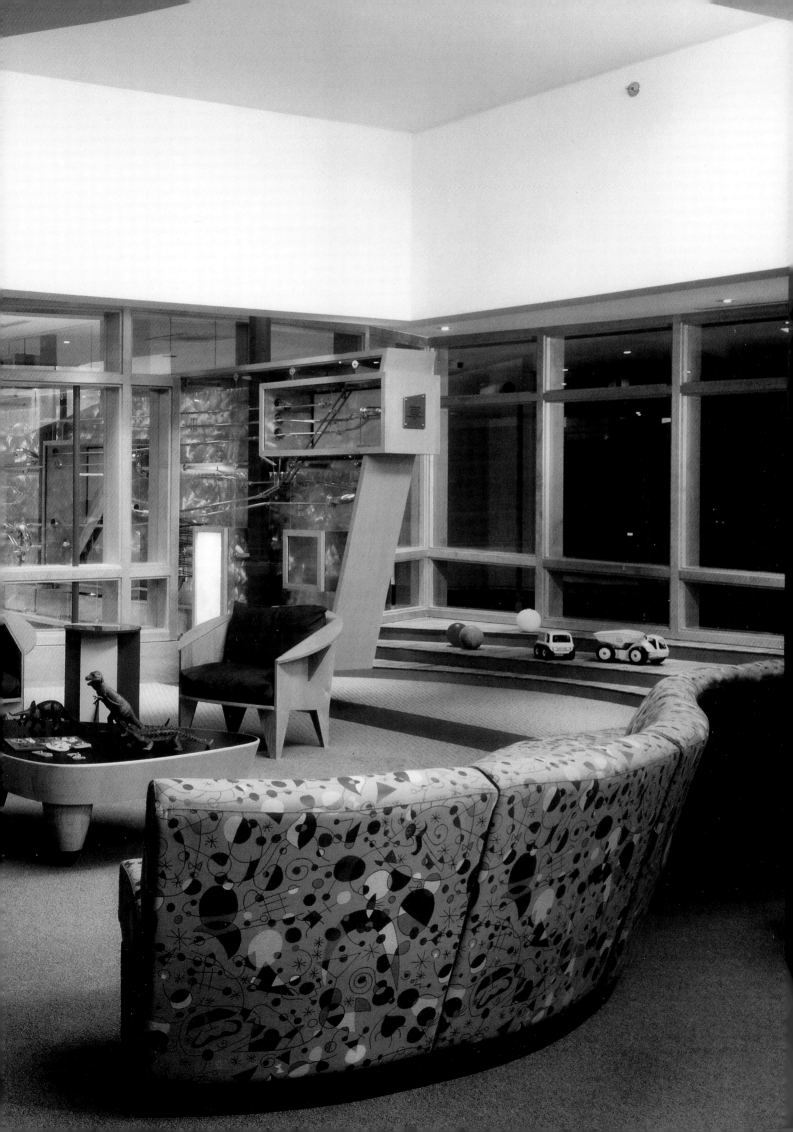

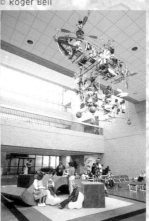

Sculpture, Texas Scottish Rite
Hospital for Children, Dallas TX
© Roger Bell

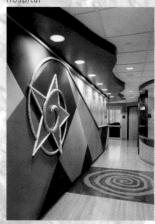

Corridor, Cardinal Glennon
Children's Hospital, St Louis MO
© Cardinal Glennon Children's
Hospital

Waiting area, Texas Scottish Rite Hospital, Dallas TX
© Roger Bell

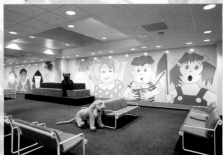

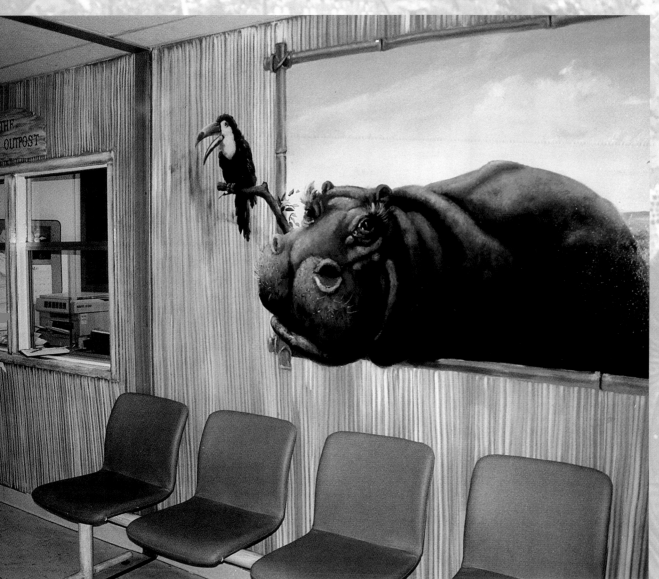

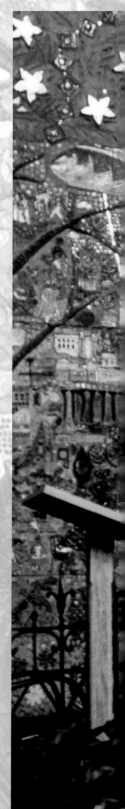

'Out of Africa', St Christopher's Hospital for Children, Philadelphia PA
© Kimberly Niemela

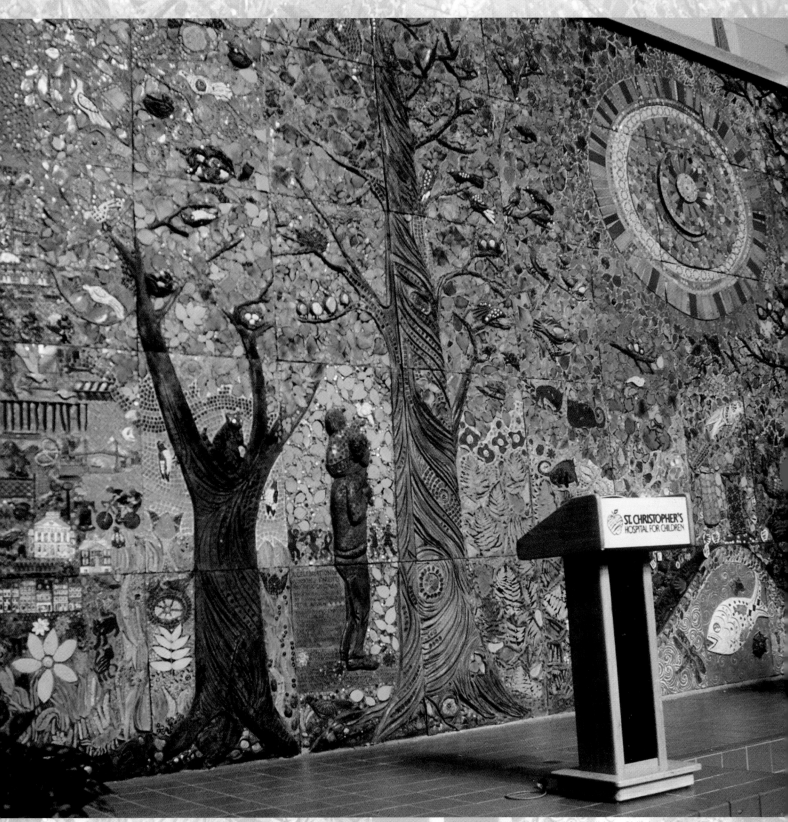

Ceramic tile wall, St Christopher's Hospital for Children, Philadelphia PA
© Kimberly Niemela

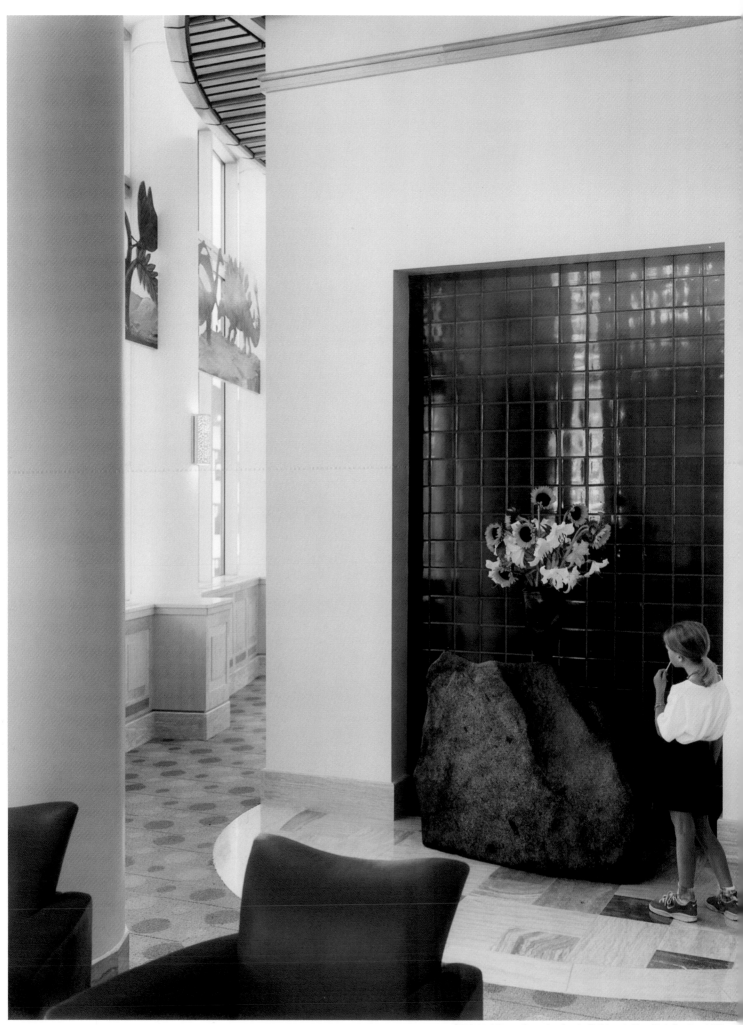

Rock sculpture, Doernbecher's Children's Hospital, Portland OR
© Eckert & Eckert

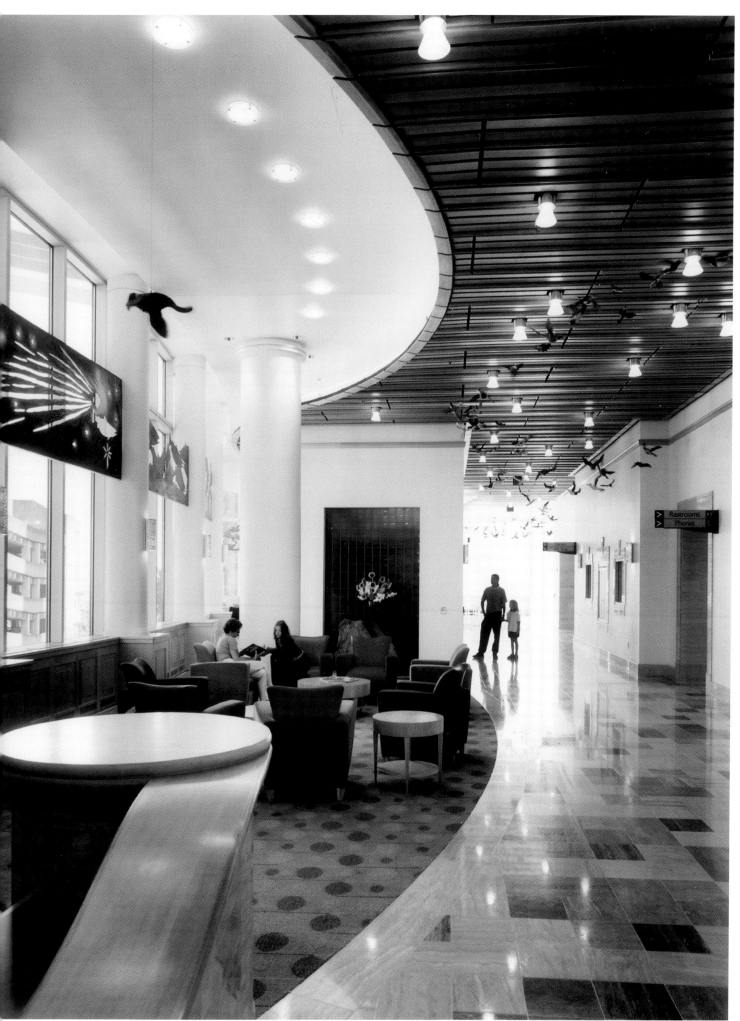

Waiting area, Doernbecher's Children's Hospital, Portland OR
© Eckert & Eckert

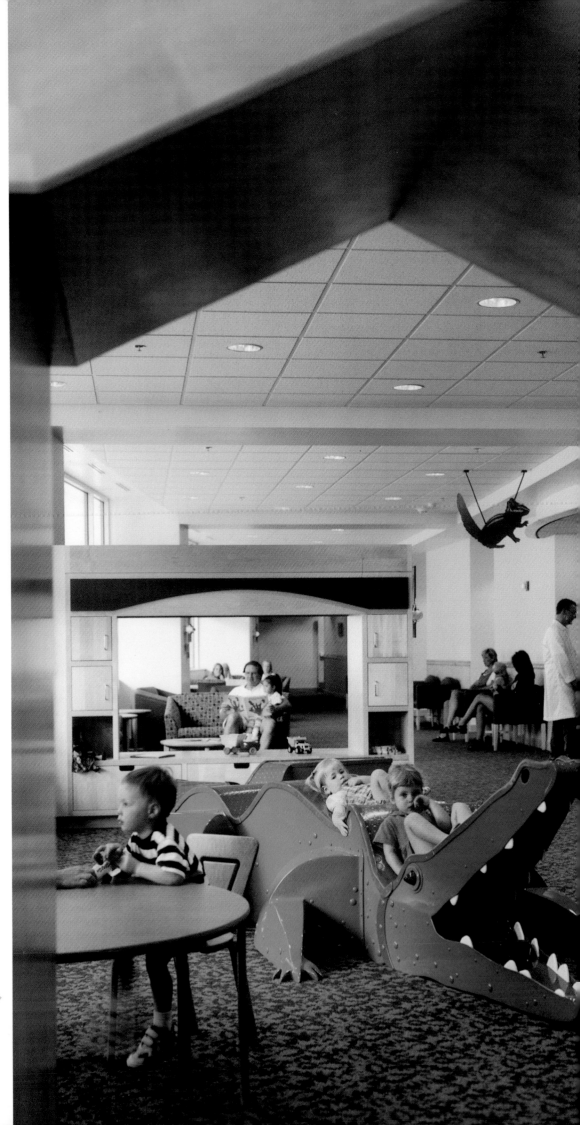

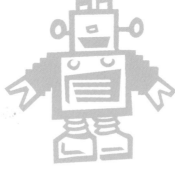

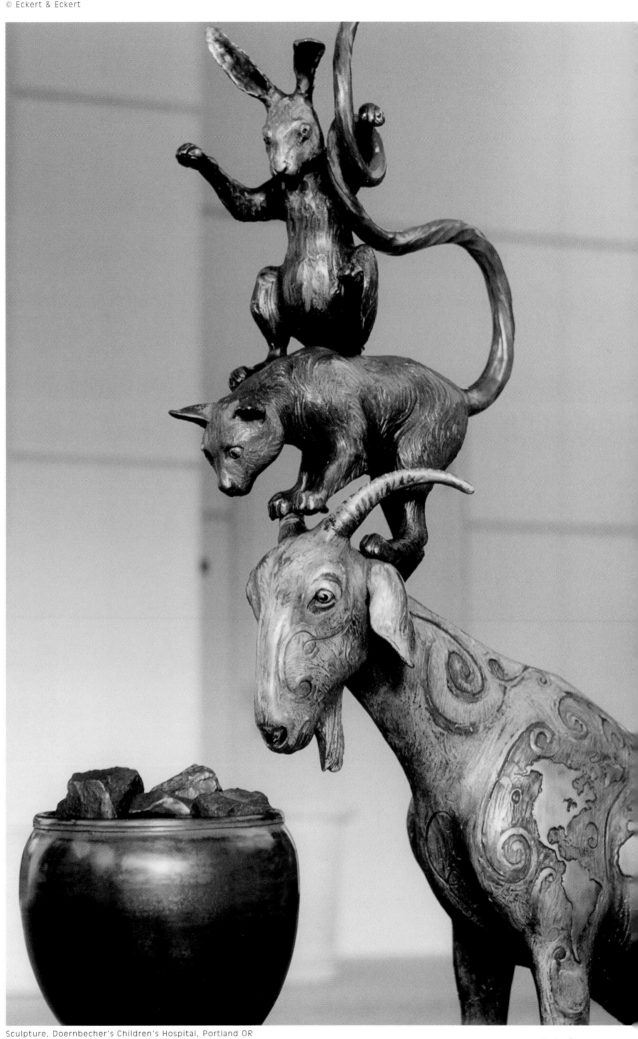

Left: Alligator sculpture, Doernbecher's Children's Hospital, Portland OR
© Eckert & Eckert

Sculpture, Doernbecher's Children's Hospital, Portland OR
© Eckert & Eckert

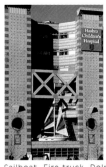 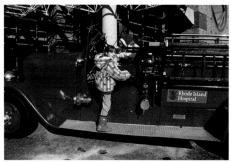 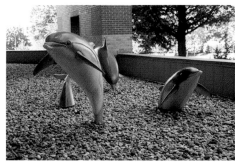

Sailboat, Fire truck, Dolphins, Hasbro Children's Hospital, Providence RI © Hasbro Children's Hospital

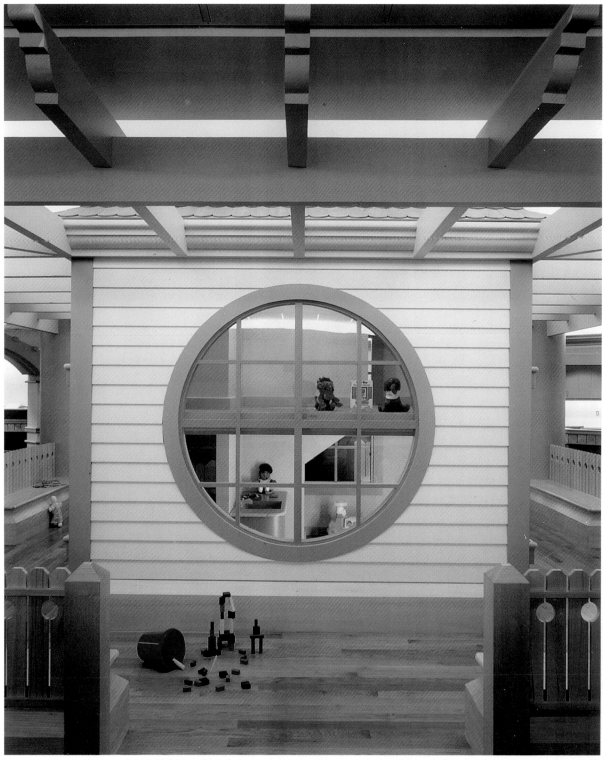

Above and right: Children's 'Club House' ambulatory waiting area, Hasbro Children's Hospital, Providence RI © Jean Smith

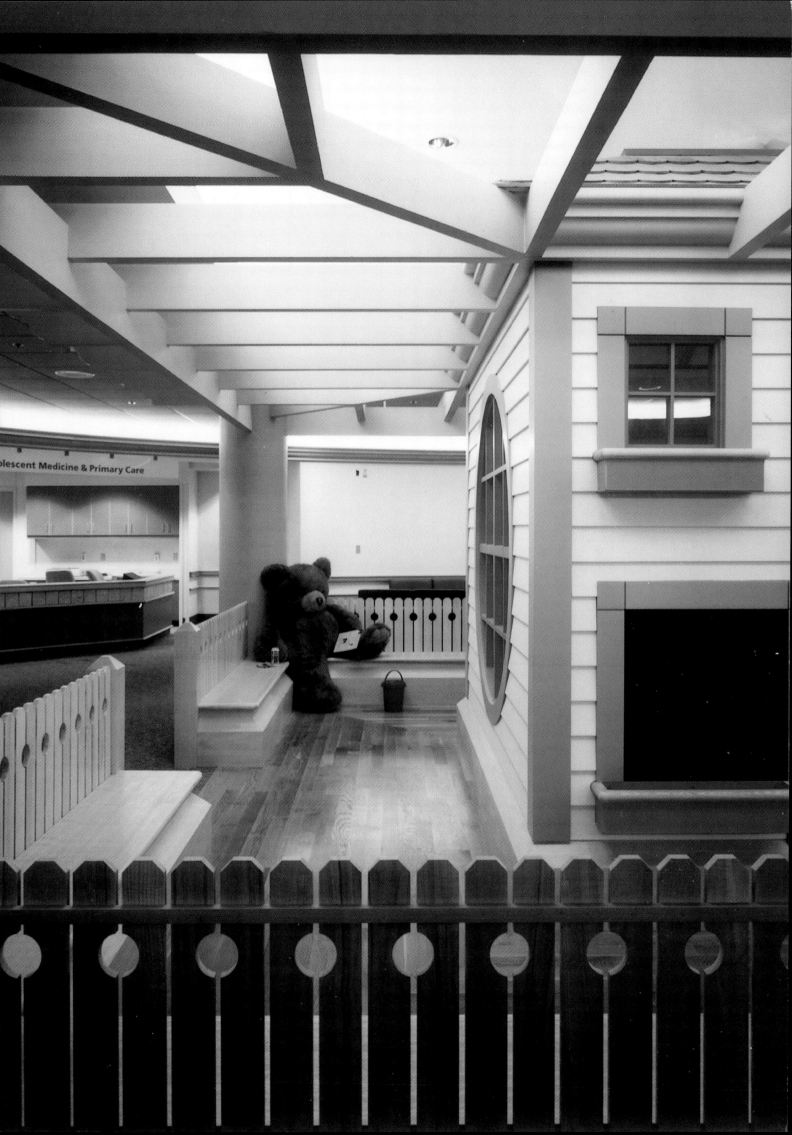

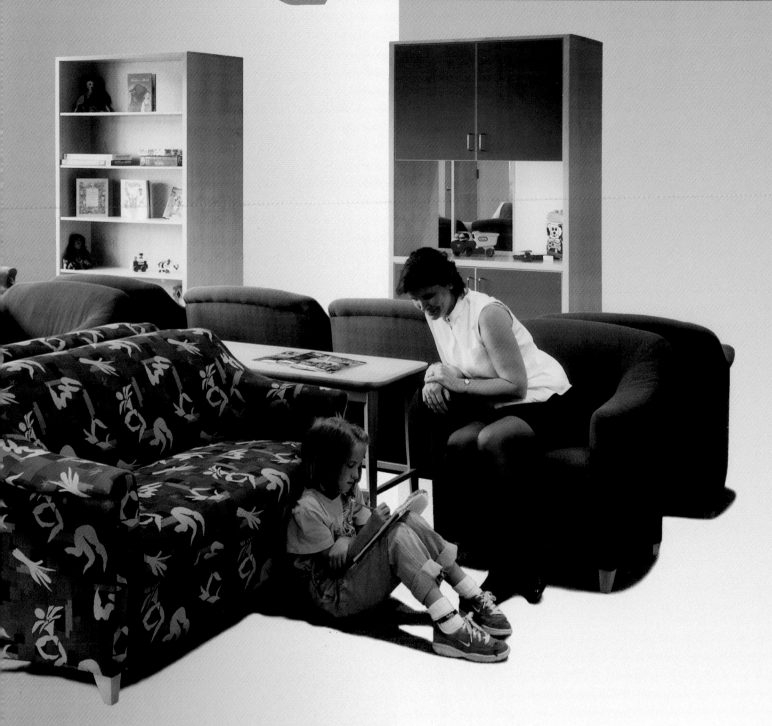

# 5 Parents as Partners

The most important element to a successful children's hospital project is the involvement of families and children in the process at the earliest stage of development. The 'Family Advisory Council' has proven to be one of the best mechanisms to start this process and create a 'family-centered' philosophy of care that starts with the design and continues through operating policy.

To assist hospitals in their efforts to include parents as partners, the Association for the Care of Children's Health has developed the following key elements:

1. Incorporating into policy and practice the recognition that the family is the constant in a child's life, while the service systems and support personnel within those systems fluctuate.

2. Facilitating family/professional collaboration at all levels of the hospital, home and community care.

3. Exchanging complete and unbiased information between families and professionals in a supportive manner at all times.

4. Incorporating into policy and practice the recognition and honoring of cultural diversity, including ethnic, racial, spiritual, social, economic, educational, emotional, and environmental, to meet the diverse needs of families.

5. Encouraging and facilitating family support and networking.

6. Ensuring that hospital, home, and community service and support systems for children needing specialized health and developmental care are flexible, accessible, and comprehensive in responding to diverse family identified needs.

7. Appreciating families as families and children as children, recognizing that they possess a wide range of strengths, concerns, emotions and aspirations beyond their need for specialized health and developmental services and support.

**Don Brunnquell, President**
Association for the Care of Children's Health

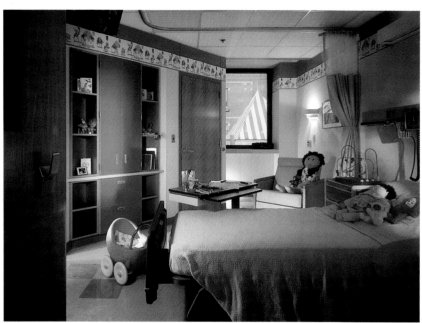

Above and below: Patient room, Children's Hospital Medical Center, Akron OH
© Scott McDonald/Hedrich-Blessing

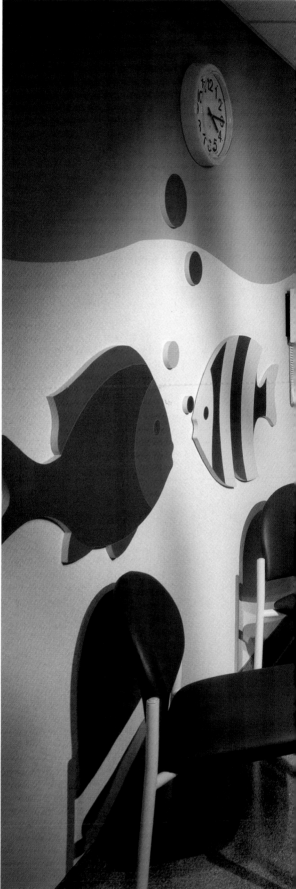

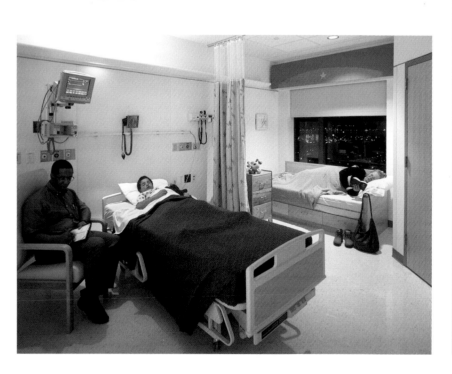

Loyola PICU patient room, Children's Hospital of the King's Daughters, Norfolk VA © Children's Hospital of the King's Daughters

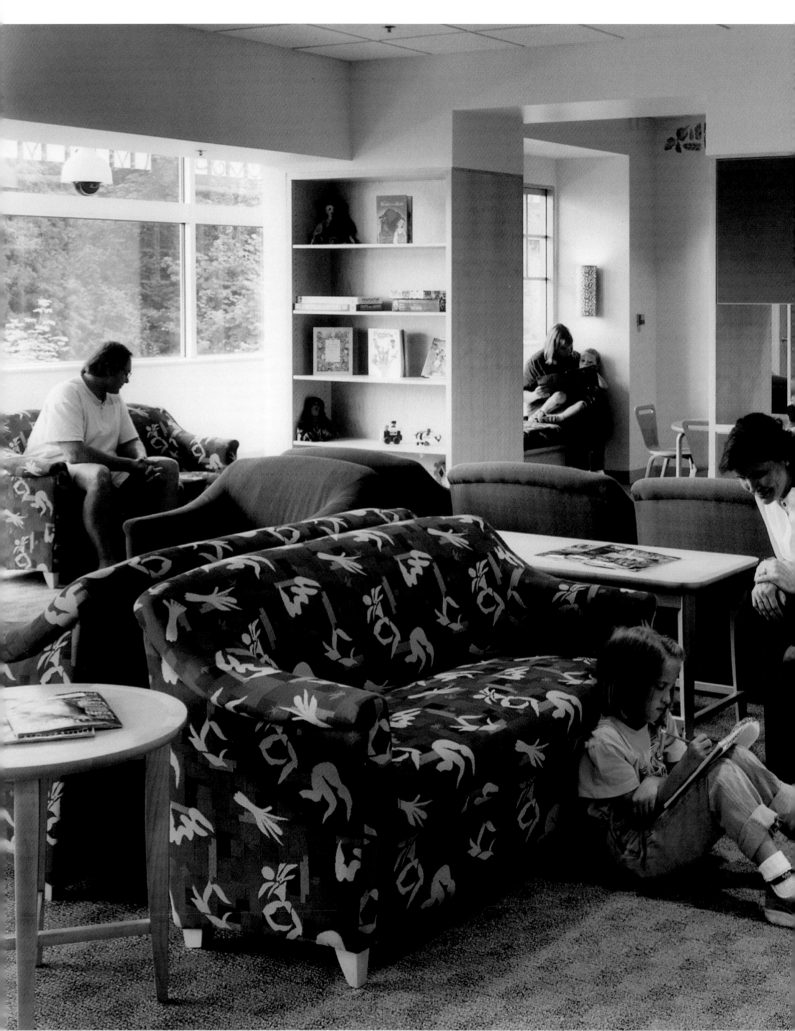

Waiting area, Doernbecher's Children's Hospital, Portland OR
© Eckert & Eckert

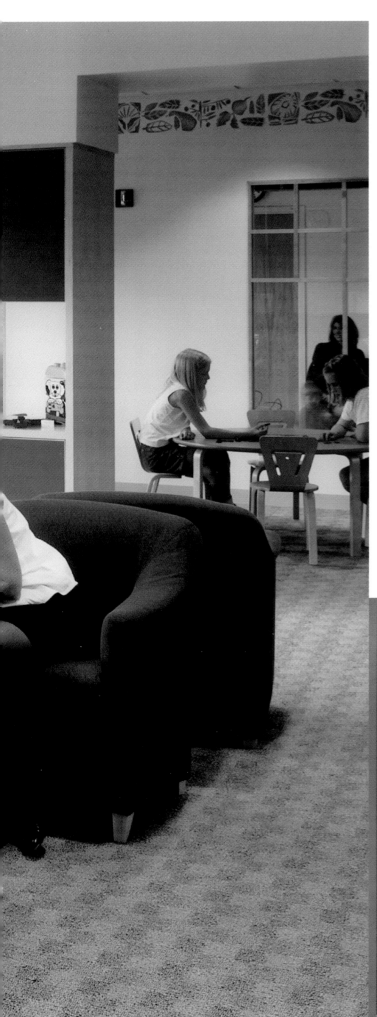

Patient room, Doernbecher's Children's Hospital, Portland OR
© Eckert & Eckert

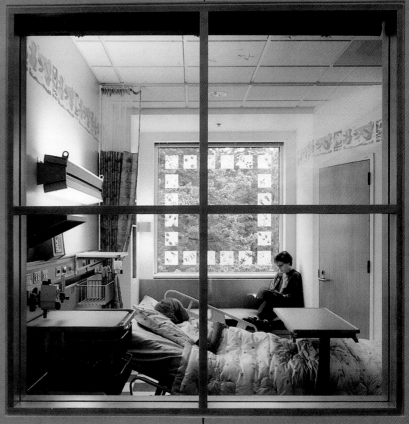

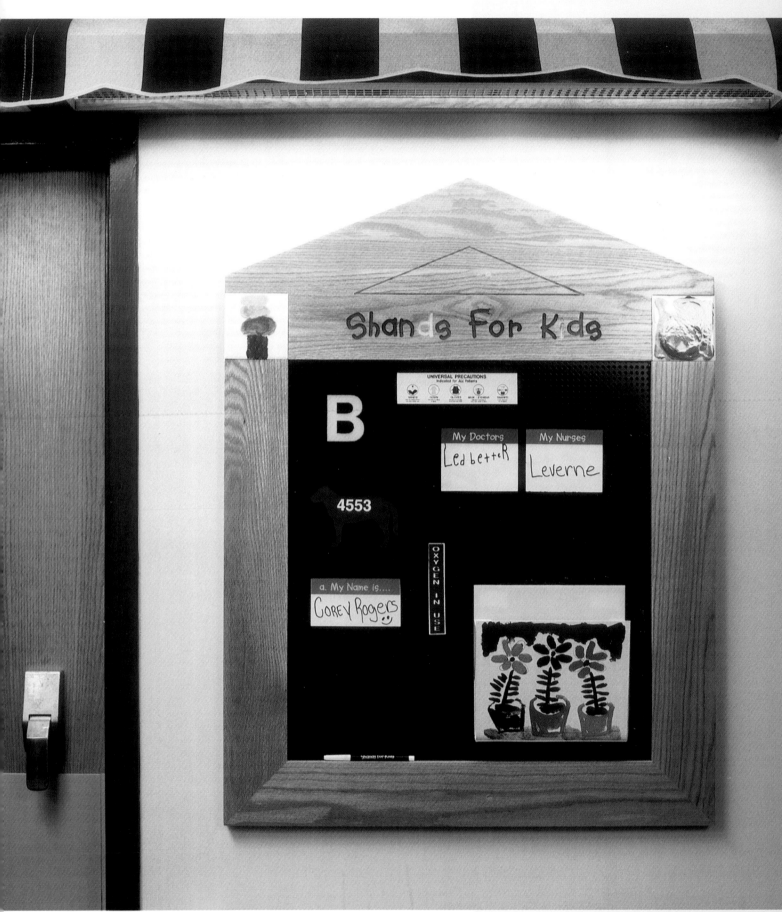

Child's personal bedroom, Shands Children's Hospital, Gainesville FL
© Shands Children's Hospital

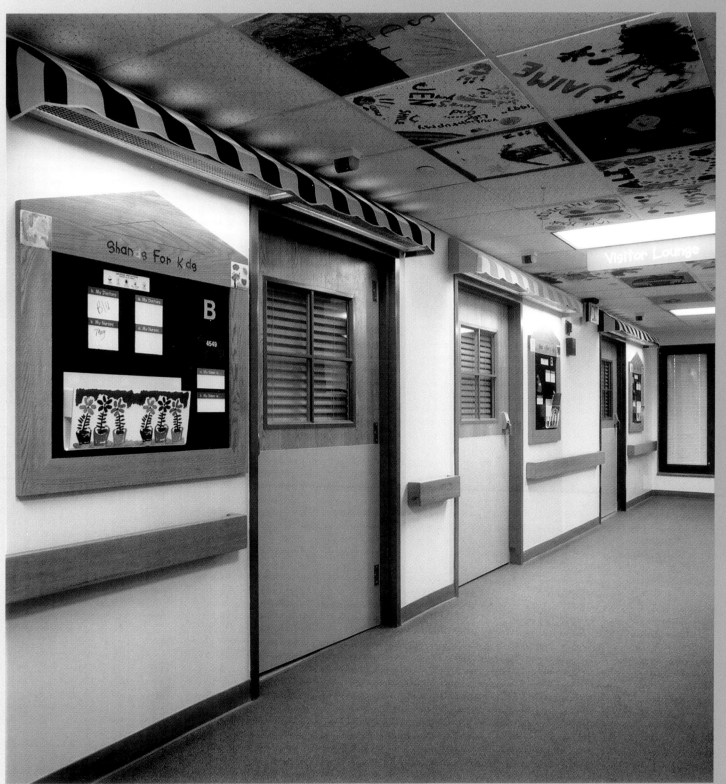

Corridor, Shands Children's Hospital, Gainesville FL

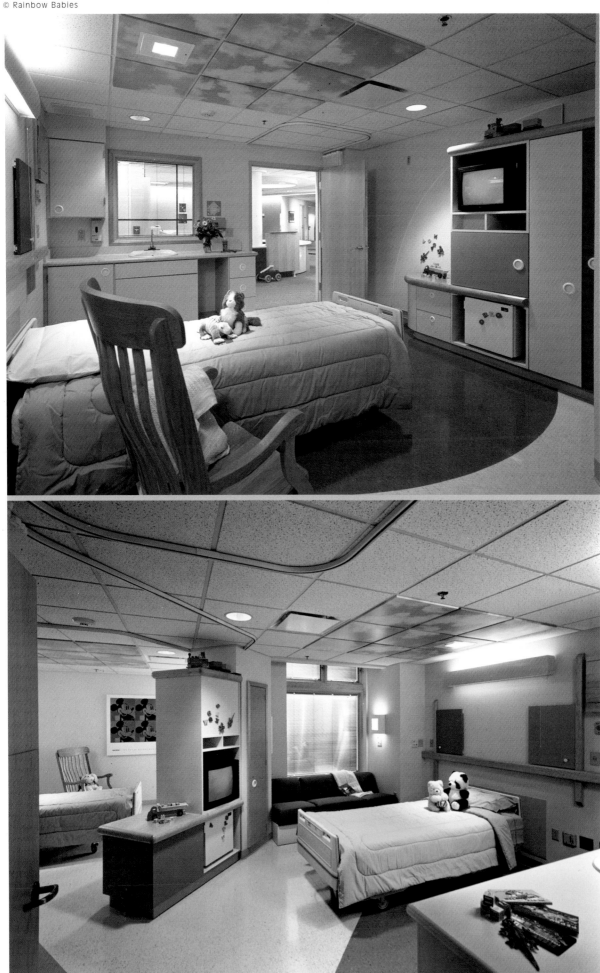

Single patient room, Rainbow Babies, Cleveland OH
© Rainbow Babies

Right: Gift shop, The Children's Hospital of Philadelphia, Philadelphia PA
© Robert Benson

Double patient room, Rainbow Babies, Cleveland OH © Rainbow Babies

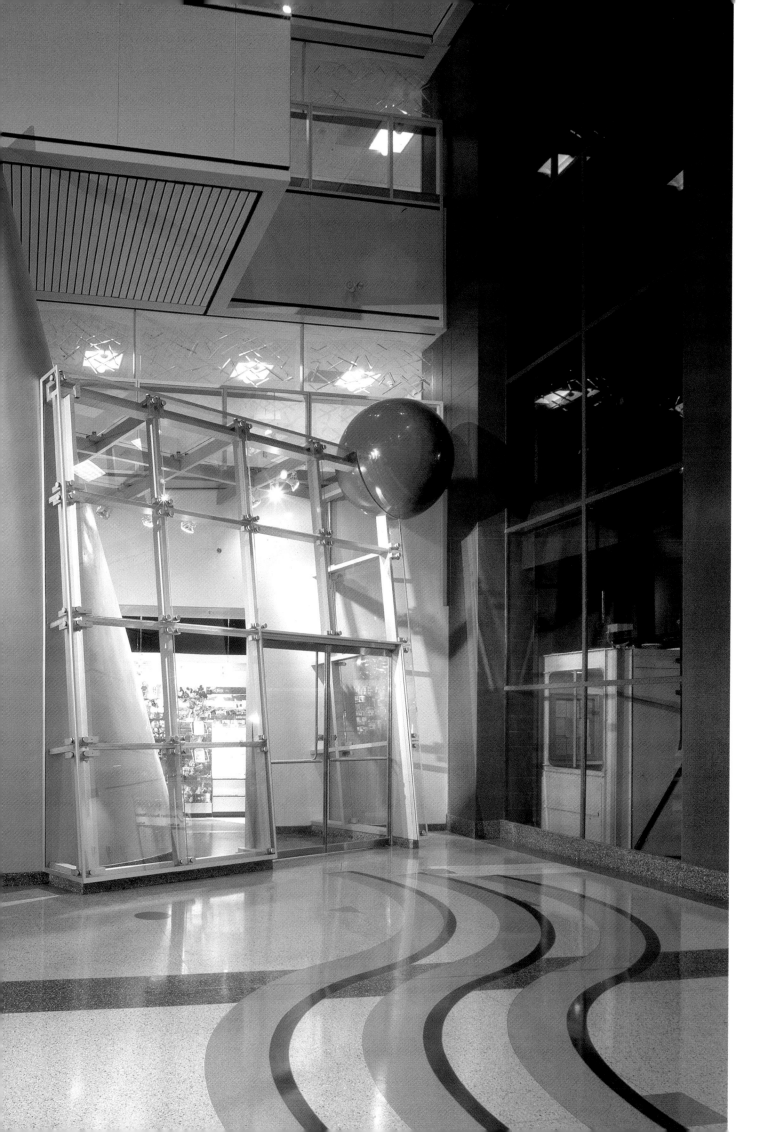

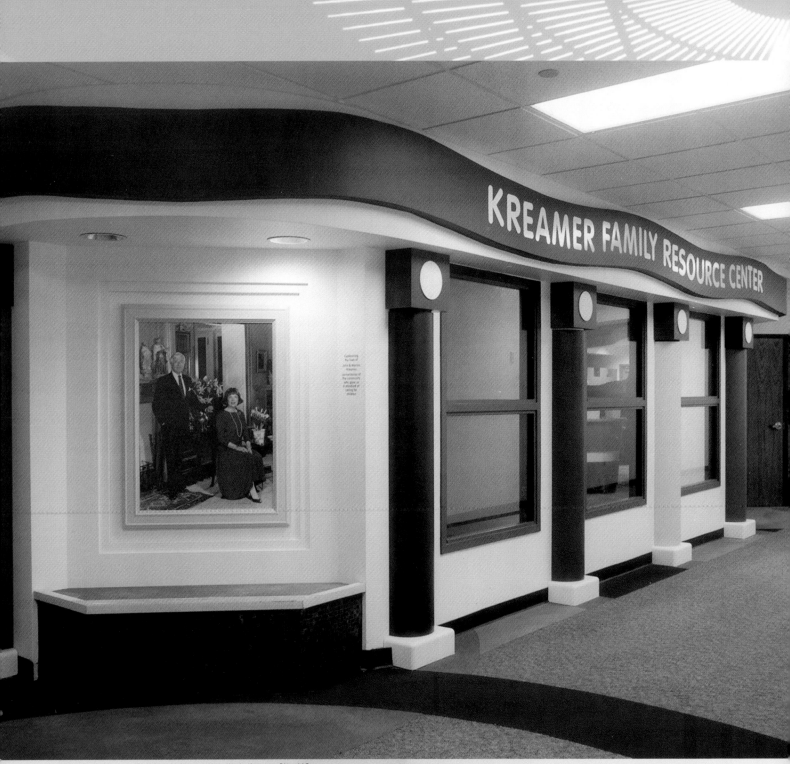

Resource Center, Children's Mercy Hospital, Kansas City MO
© Bruce Mathews

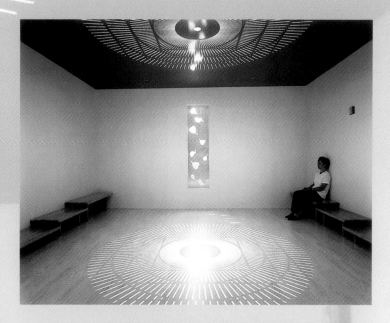

Meditation room, Doernbecher's Children's Hospital, Portland OR
© Eckert & Eckert

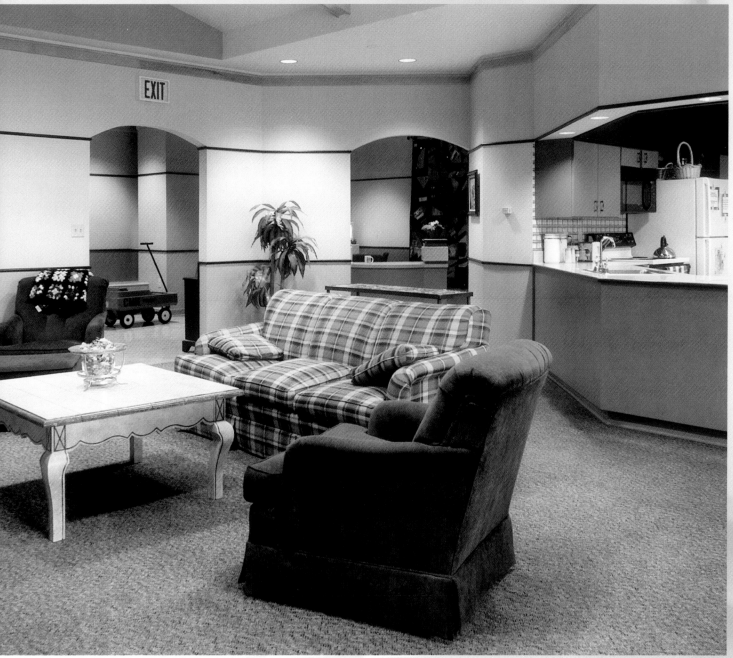

Family room, Children's Mercy Hospital, Kansas City MO
© Bruce Mathews

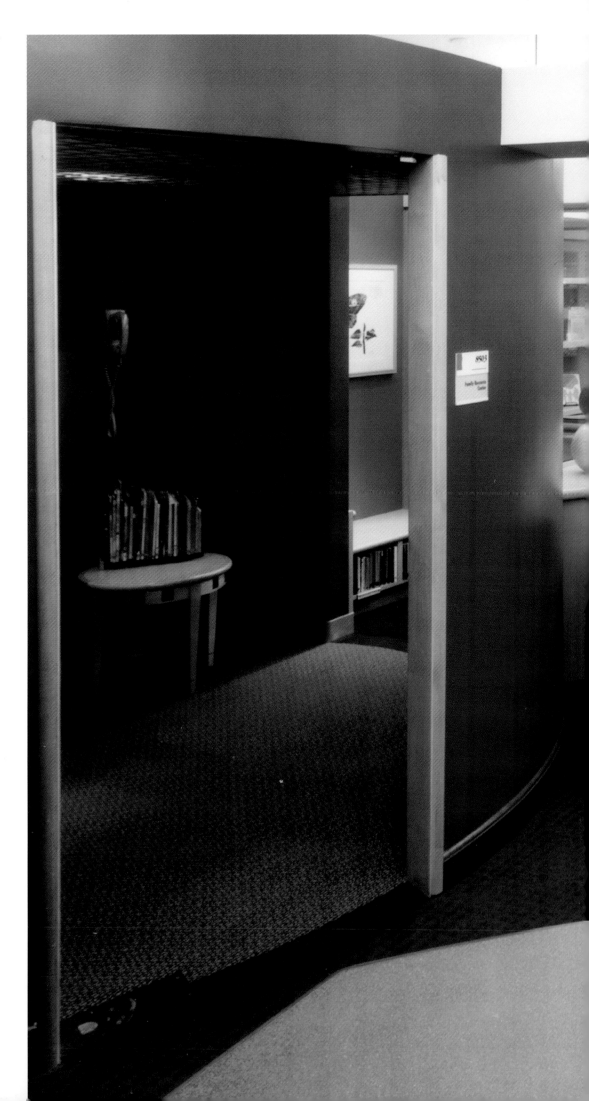

'Family Library' at The Connelly
Resource Center for Families,
The Children's Hospital of
Philadelphia, Philadelphia PA
© Feinknopf

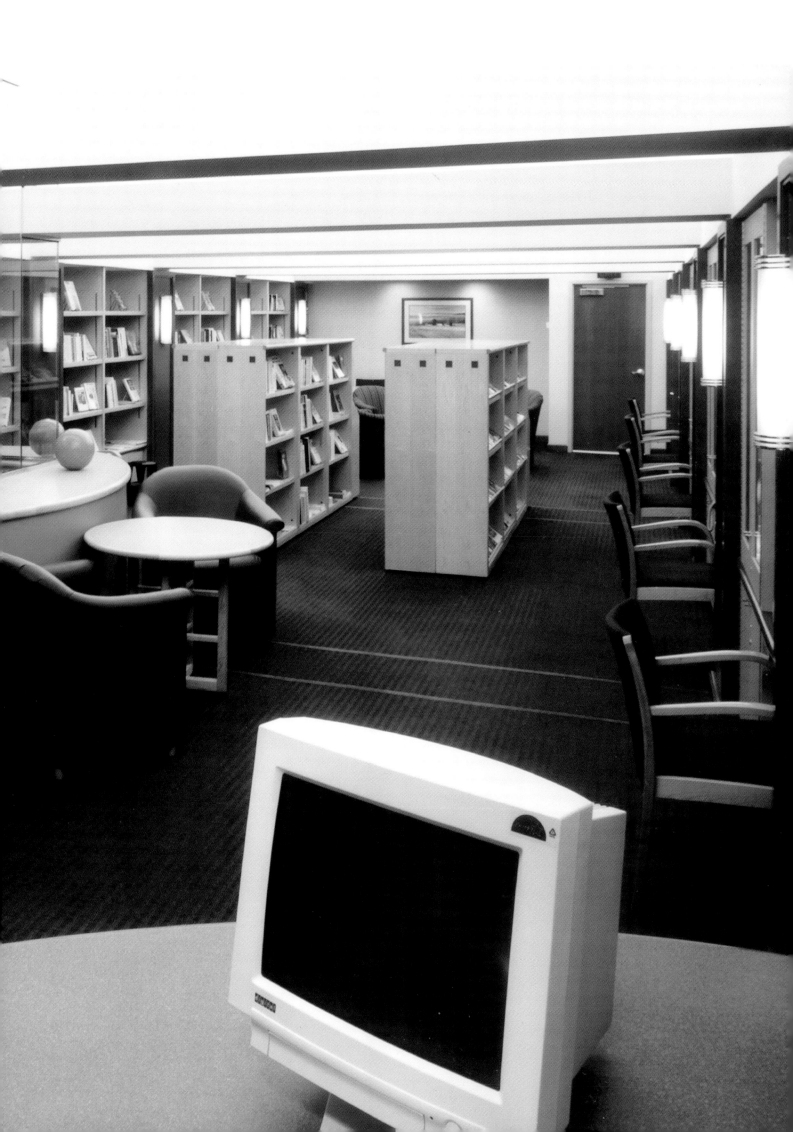

Patient room showing parent's sleep couch, The Children's Hospital of Philadelphia, Philadelphia PA
© Robert Benson

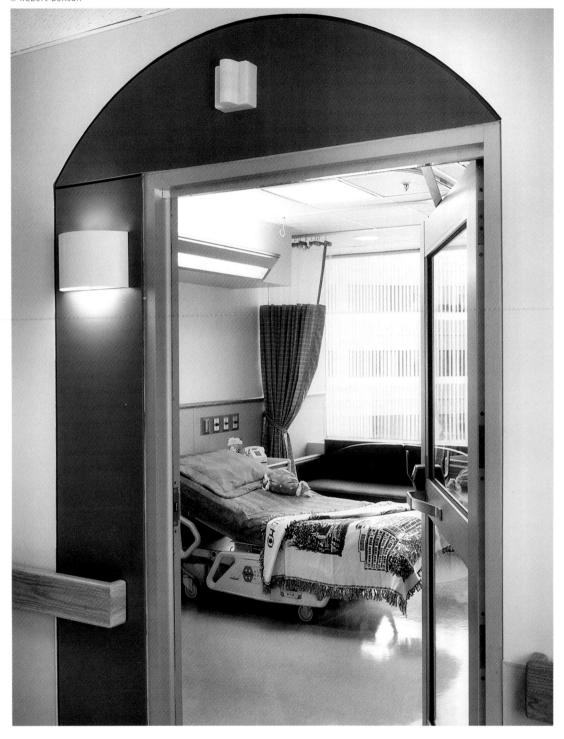

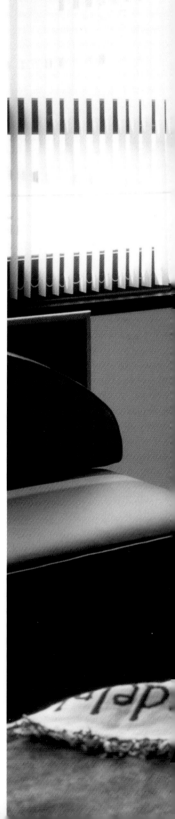

Patient room showing custom cabinetry, The Children's Hospital of Philadelphia, Philadelphia PA
© Robert Benson

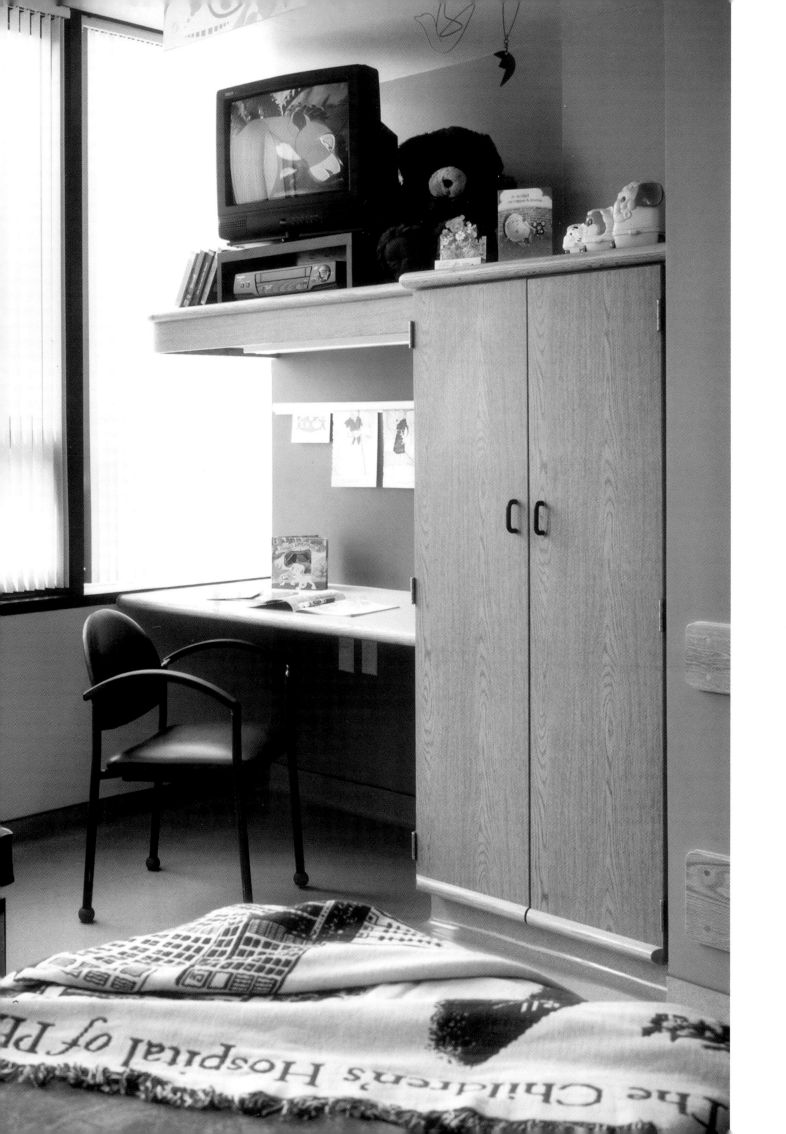

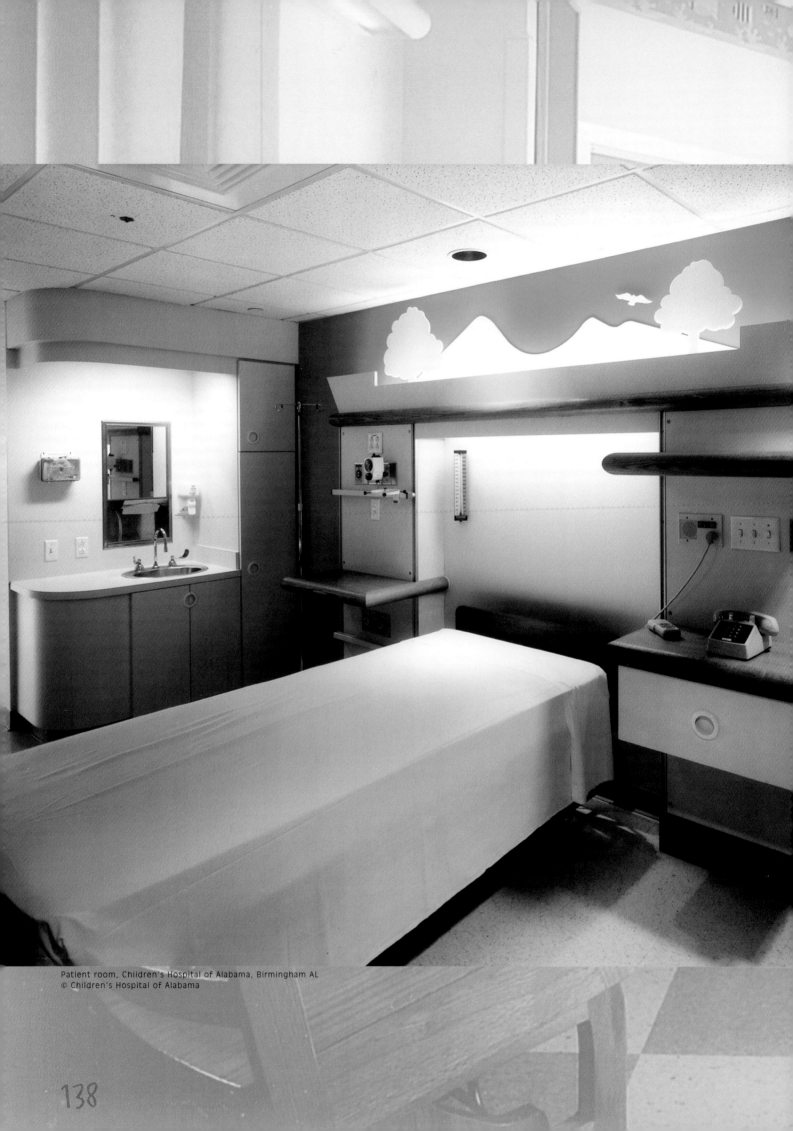

Patient room, Children's Hospital of Alabama, Birmingham AL
© Children's Hospital of Alabama

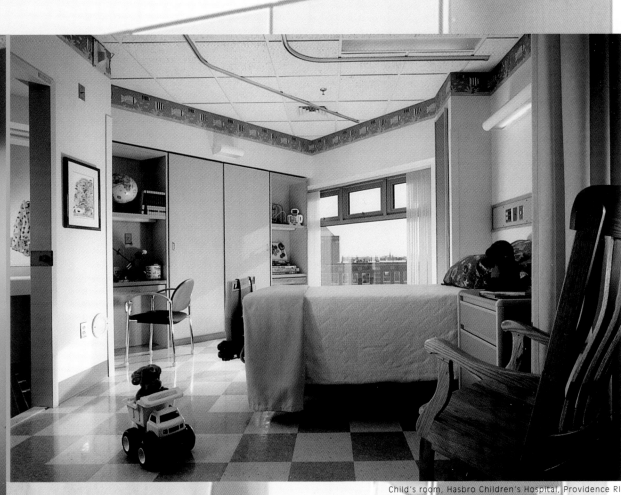

Child's room, Hasbro Children's Hospital, Providence RI
© Robert Miller

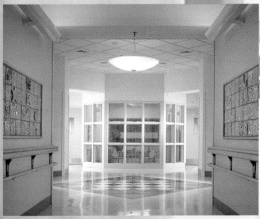

Parents' lounge, Hasbro Children's Hospital,
Providence RI © Robert Miller

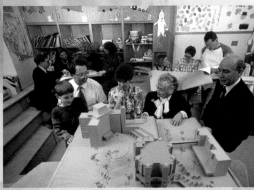

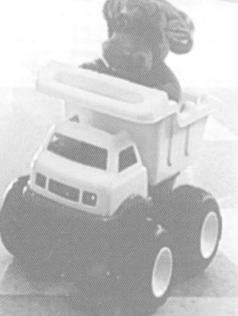

Family Advisory Council,
Hasbro Children's Hospital, Providence RI
© Lou Trombetti

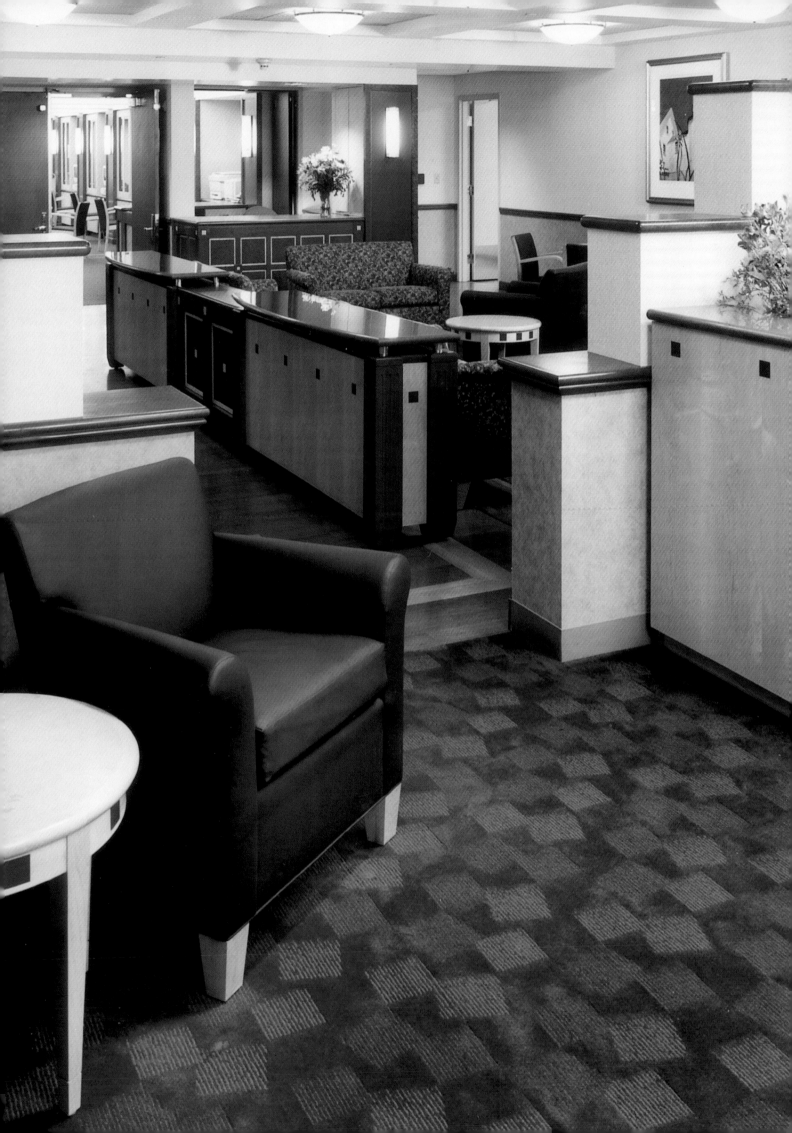

Family lounge at The Connelly Resource Center for Families,
The Children's Hospital of Philadelphia, Philadelphia PA
© Feinknopf

Child's room, Valley Children's Hospital, Madera CA
© Kelly Peterson

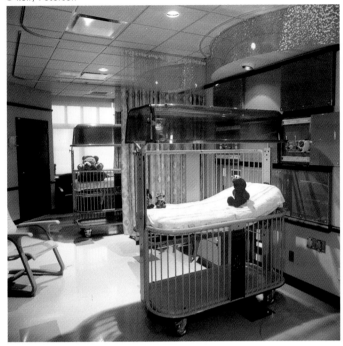

Food court, Valley Children's Hospital, Madera CA
© Kelly Peterson

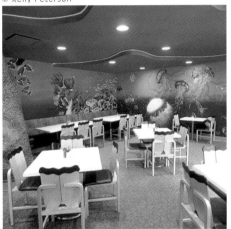

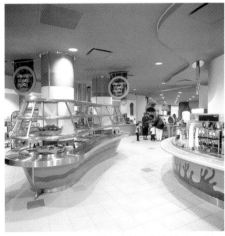

Food court, Valley Children's Hospital, Madera CA
© Kelly Peterson

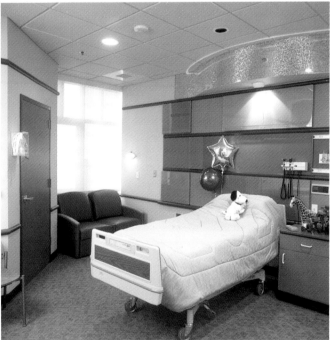

Child's room, Valley Children's Hospital, Madera CA
© Kelly Peterson

Following pages:
Food court, Children's Hospital and Health Center, San Diego CA
© Children's Hospital and Health Center

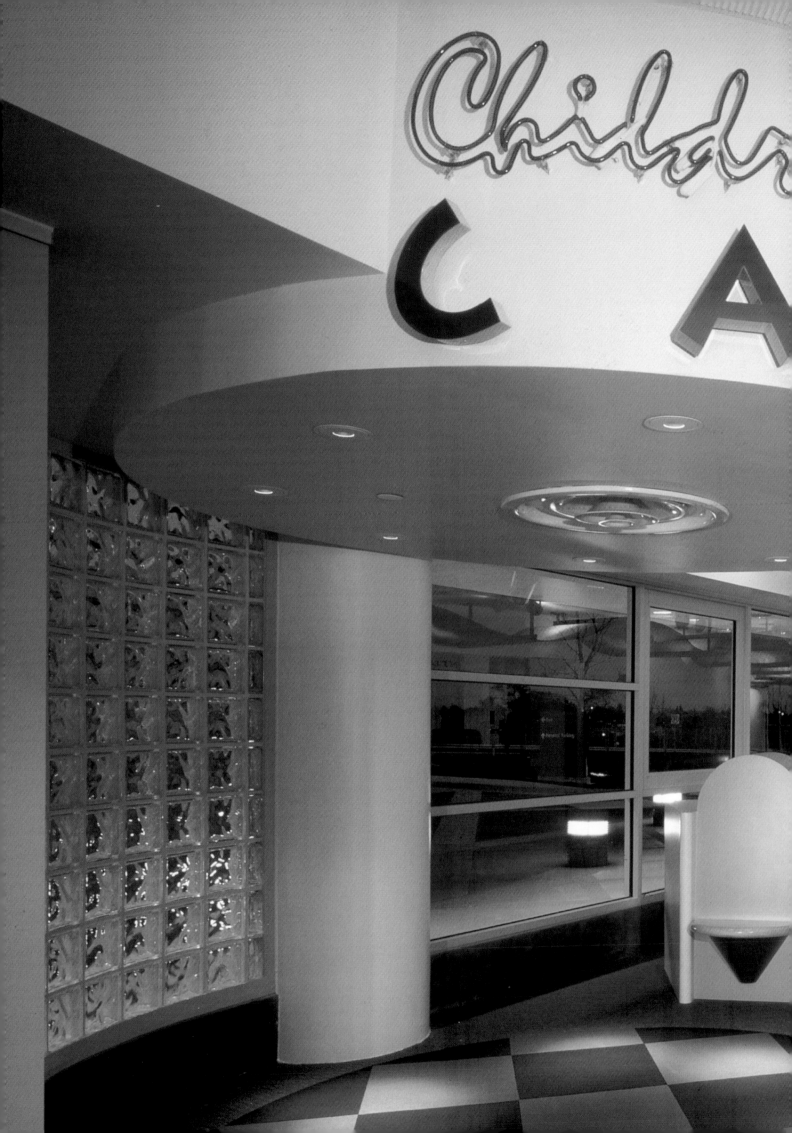

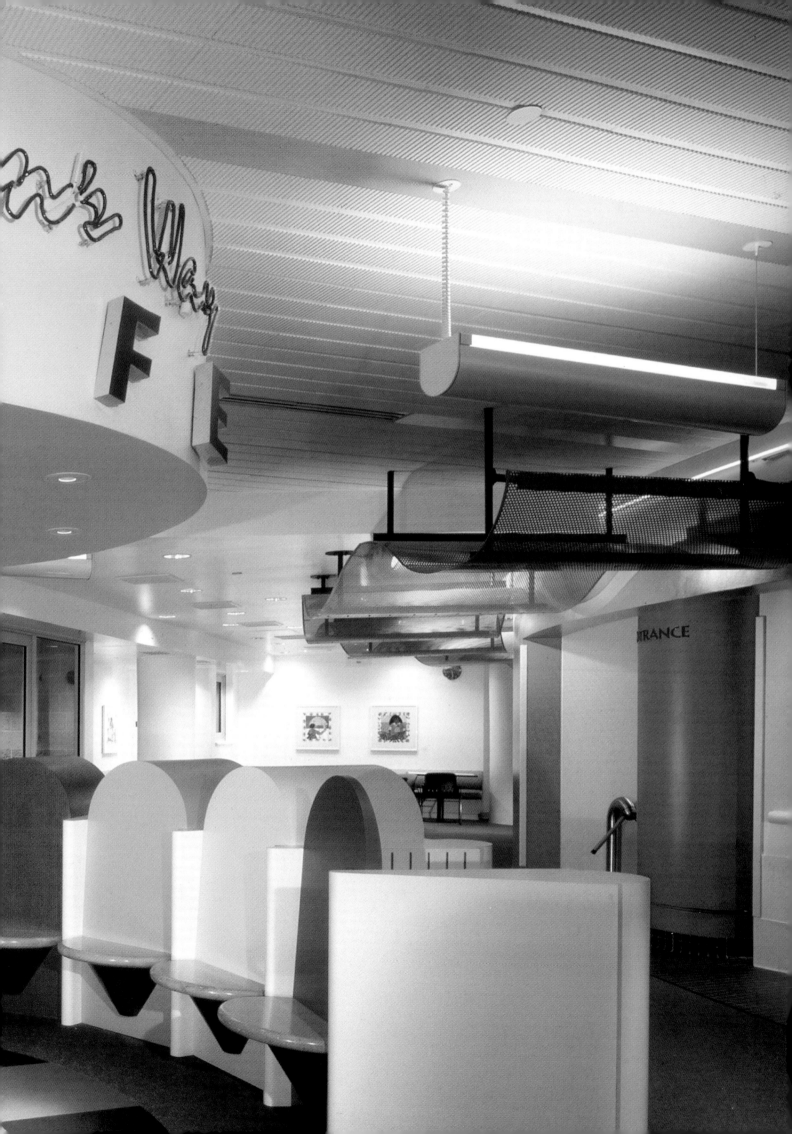

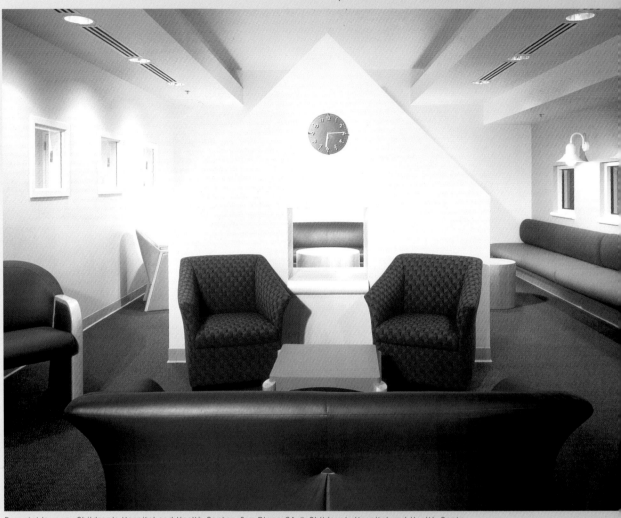

Parents' lounge, Children's Hospital and Health Center, San Diego CA © Children's Hospital and Health Center

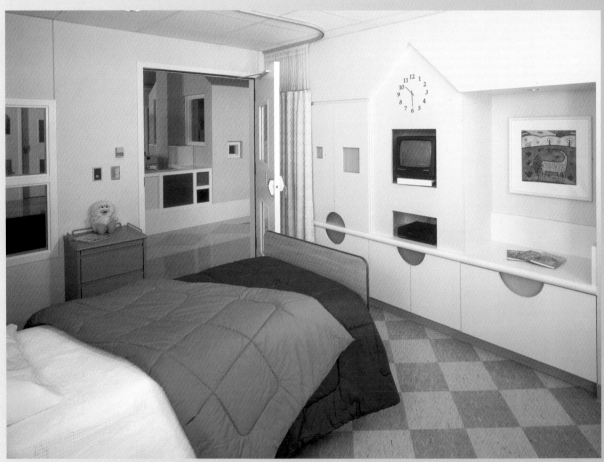

Patient room, Children's Hospital and Health Center, San Diego CA © Children's Hospital and Health Center

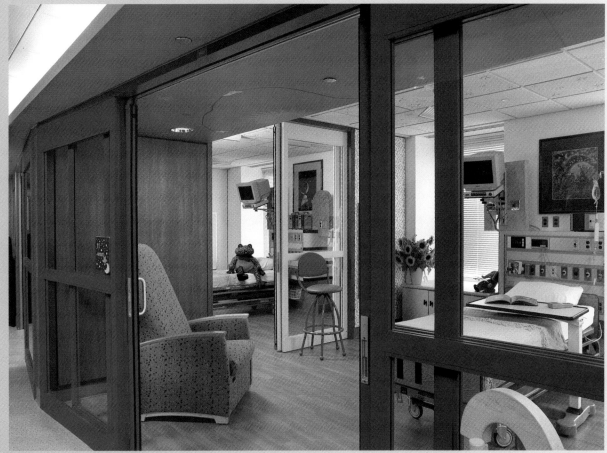

PICU room, Babies & Children's Hospital at New York Presbyterian, New York NY
© Colin McRae

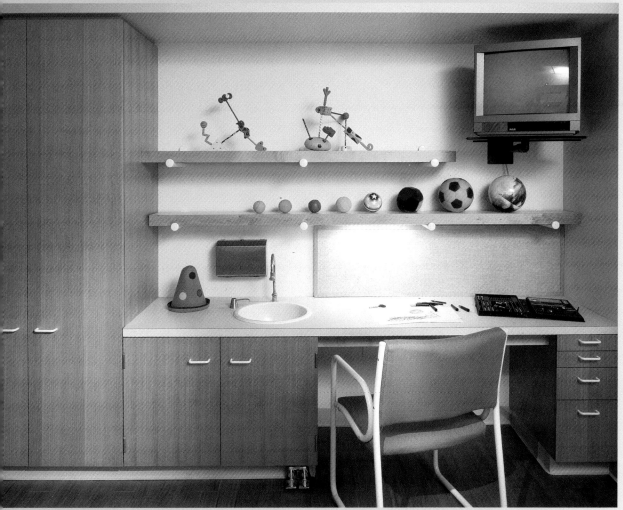

Patient room, Lucile Salter Packard Children's Hospital, Palo Alto CA © Lucile Salter Packard Children's Hospital

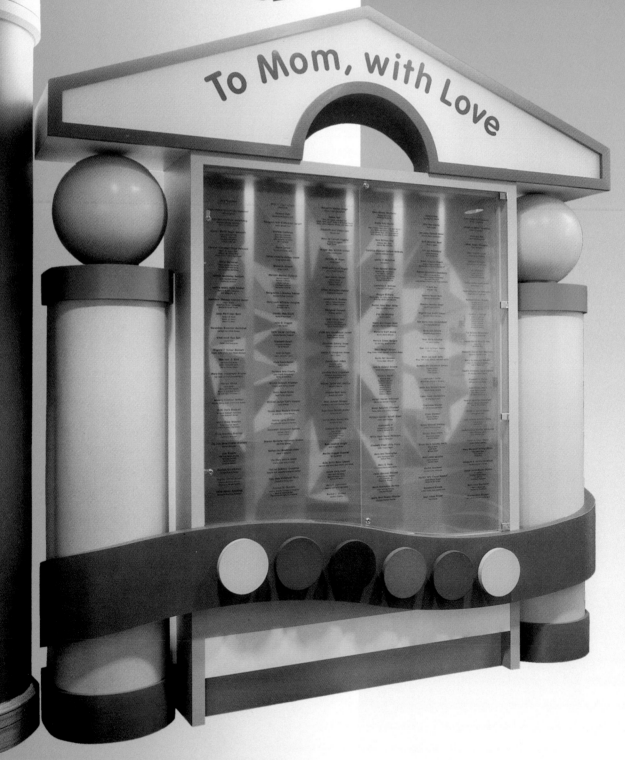

# 6

# The Importance of Marketing and Communication

To Mom, with Love

The creation of a new facility is an outstanding opportunity to significantly enhance the overall image of the entire hospital within the community. To maximize this opportunity as well as ensure the success of the project, every effort must be made to involve all constituencies from both the hospital and the community. These constituencies include: parents, patients, schools, civic groups, the art community, the police/ambulance/fire departments, and the Family Advisory Council, to name just a few. Their participation should involve both fund-raising as well as input into the program. Don't forget that staff, parents and patients are key communicators of messages for the hospital.

The more creative the project team becomes in looking for opportunities to involve the community in all stages of the project, the greater the level of overall success. These opportunities include the traditional milestones of a project, i.e. ground-breaking, 'topping off' (highest piece of steel put in place), public open houses and tours, creation of a mascot, and the use of celebrities to publicize the project. Very successful projects go beyond the usual and have included such events as, the 'Wrong Trousers Day' (from the Oscar winning film characters Wallace and Grommet) held in Bristol, England, or a 'Barn Raising' held to build the pre-construction building at Westchester Medical Center, Valhalla NY. Consider making all these events unique and unlike any other of its kind ever experienced in the region.

Recognize that children's hospitals are the 'jewels in the crown' of a healthcare system and maximize the 'halo effect' that they will produce. This effect can be quantified to include increased market share, significant increases in philanthropy, enhanced ability to recruit staff and volunteers, and a significant impact on the overall hospital's image in the community. The hospital will benefit long term from the involvement of the community from the outset.

Last, but most important, use every possible mechanism to communicate both internally and externally about your plans and the project. Never assume that you have done enough. Communicate, communicate, communicate.

**Graham Nix and David Hughes M.D.**
United Bristol Healthcare NHS Trust
Bristol, England

Prince Charles visits Royal Hospital for Sick Children, Bristol, England © Royal Hospital for Sick Children

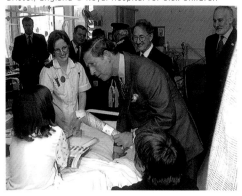

Wallace and Grommet, Royal Hospital for Sick Children, Bristol, England © Royal Hospital for Sick Children

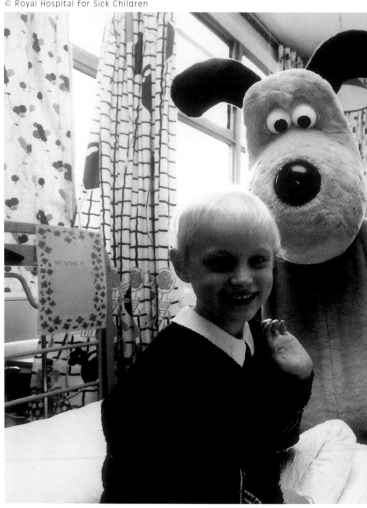

'Three Peaks in Three Days', Royal Hospital for Sick Children, Bristol, England © Royal Hospital for Sick Children

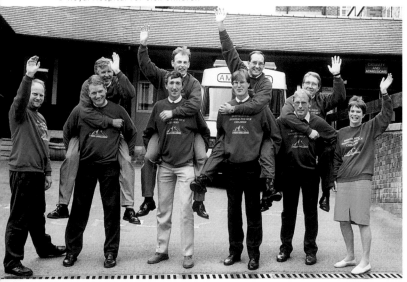

'Wrong Trousers Day', Royal Hospital for Sick Children, Bristol, England © Royal Hospital for Sick Children

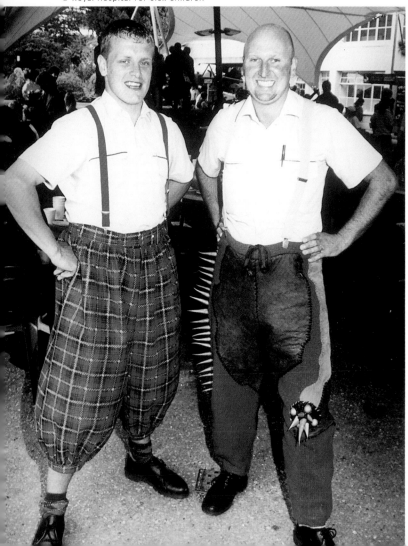

Time capsule, Royal Hospital for Sick Children, Bristol, England © Royal Hospital for Sick Children

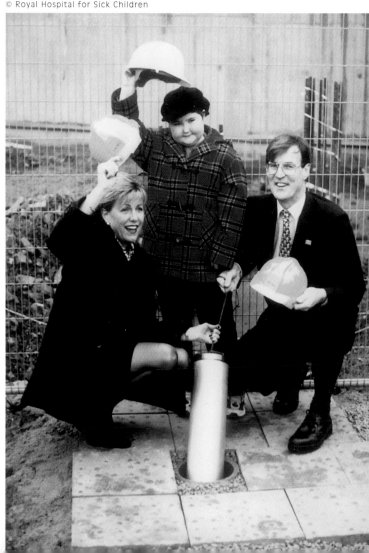

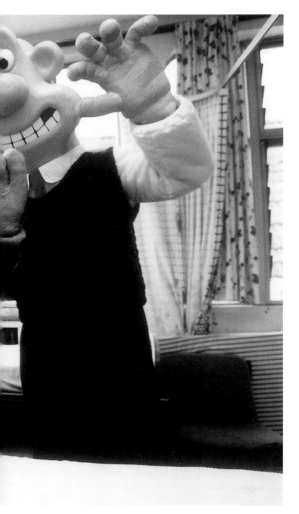

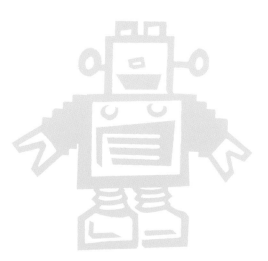

Hasbro mascot, Hasbro Children's Hospital, Providence RI © Hasbro Children's Hospital

'Miss America Ground-breaking', Hasbro Children's Hospital, Providence RI © Hasbro Children's Hospital

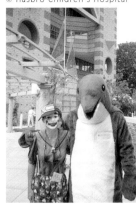

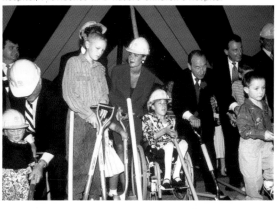

'Wrong Trousers Day', Royal Hospital for Sick Children, Bristol, England © Royal Hospital for Sick Children

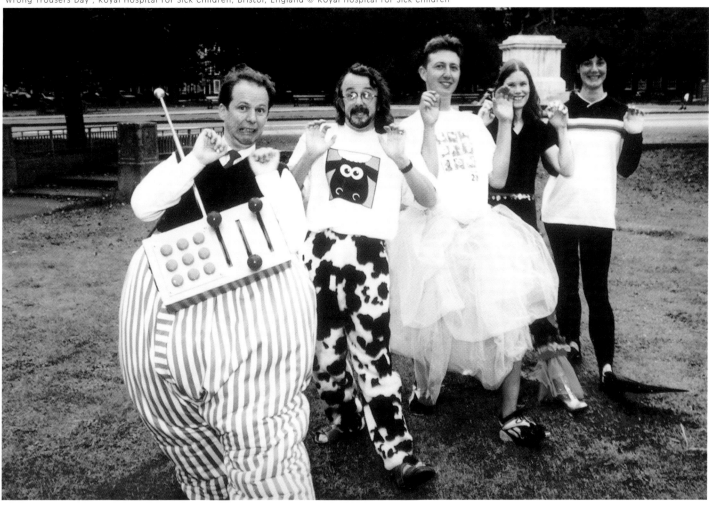

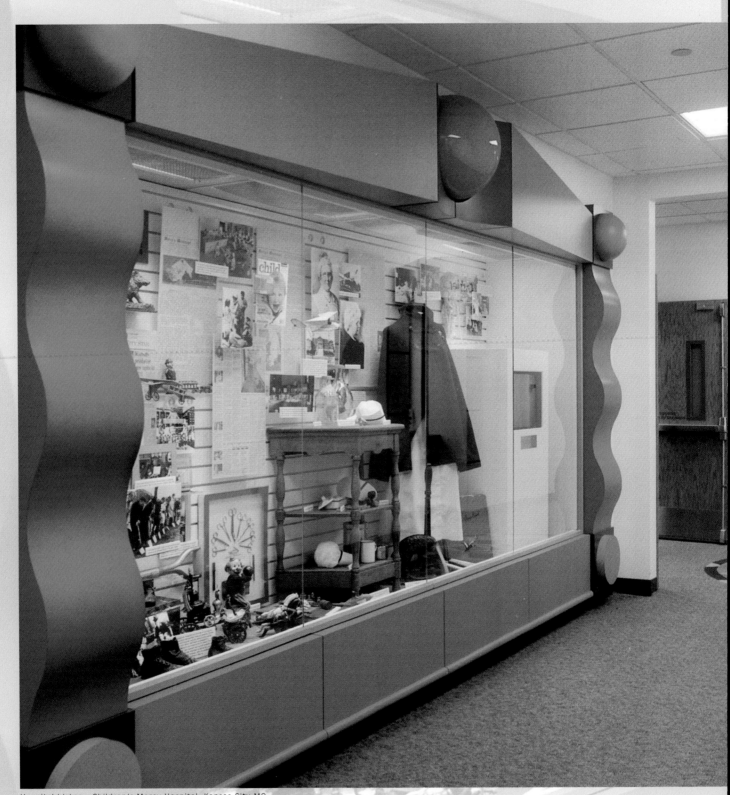

Hospital history, Children's Mercy Hospital, Kansas City MO
© Bruce Mathews

150

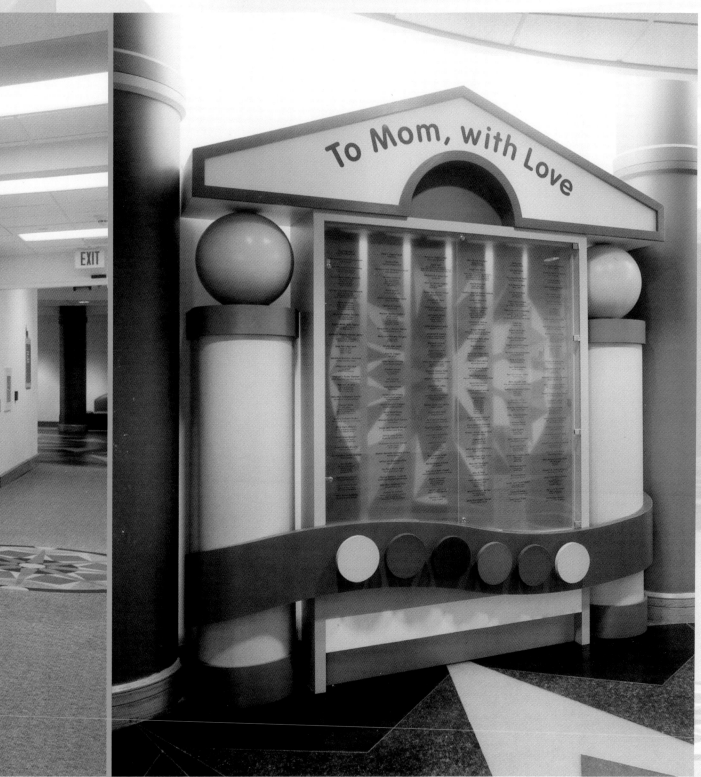

'To Mom, with Love', Children's Mercy Hospital, Kansas City MO
© Bruce Mathews

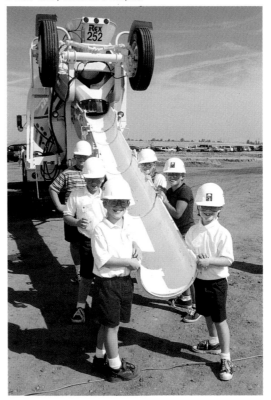

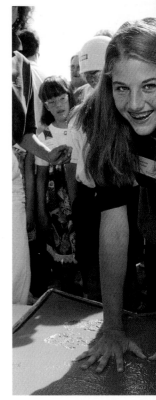

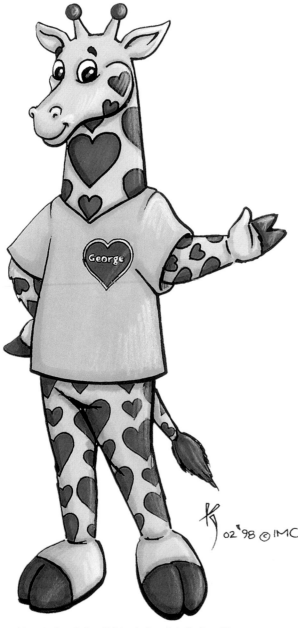

Mascot, New Valley Children's Hospital, Madera CA
Rendering © IMC

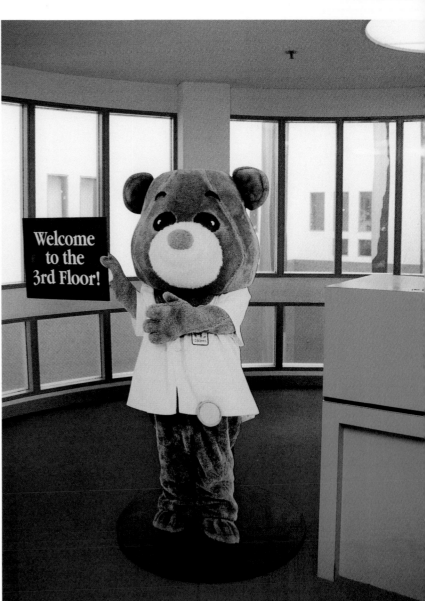

Bear Mascot, Children's National Medical Center, Washington D.C.

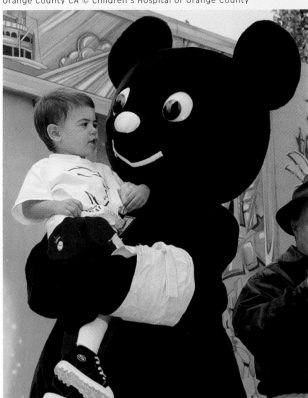

Choco Bear, Mascot, Children's Hospital of Orange County,
Orange County CA © Children's Hospital of Orange County

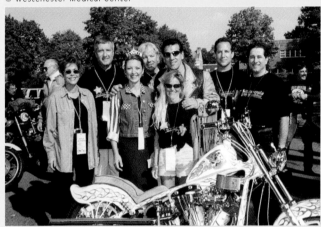

Motorcycle party, Westchester Medical Center, Valhalla NY
© Westchester Medical Center

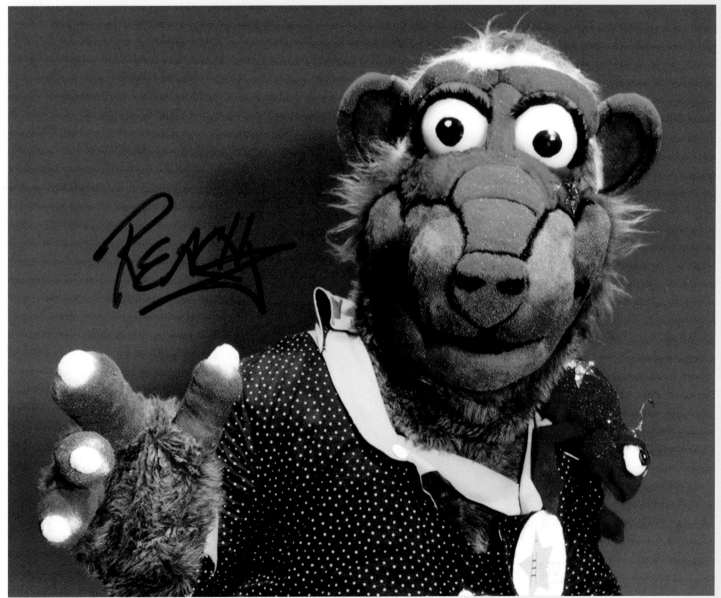

'Reach', Mascot for Maria Fareri Children's Hospital, Westchester Medical Center, Valhalla NY © Maria Fareri Children's Hospital

# 7

# The Future of Children's Healthcare Design

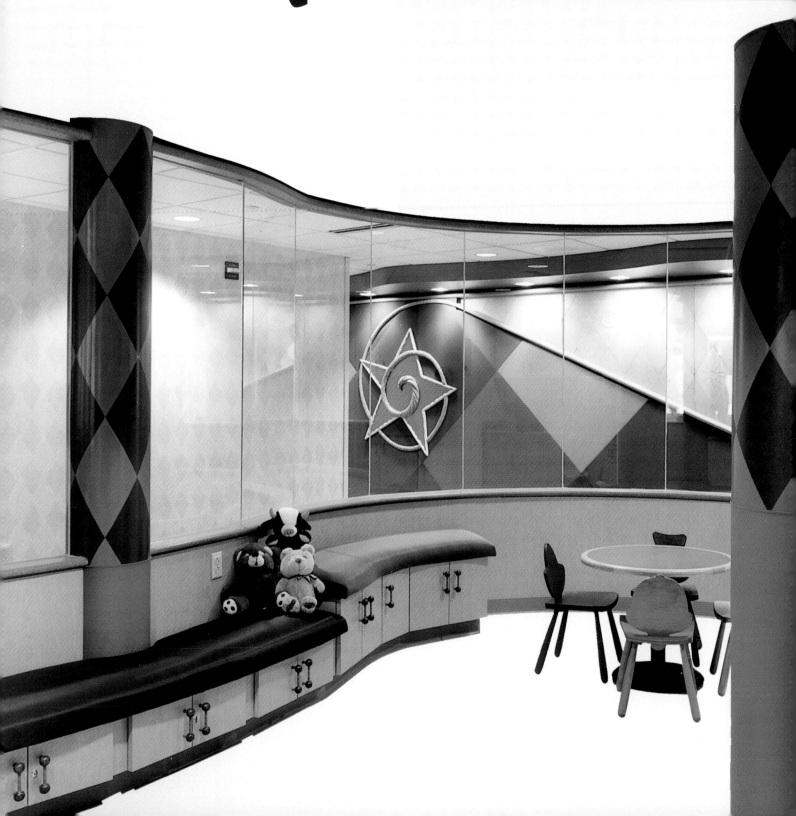

The future will bring both new challenges and new innovations to children's care. The presence of more acutely ill children in hospitals will force the need for more intensive medical environments. Financial pressures will continue to demand more efficient operations. Healthcare environments will respond to these challenges with more accommodating and comforting places for children and their families. Buildings scaled to children, accommodations for personal control and privacy, intuitive wayfinding, and family-friendly facilities will become the norm. In addition to the many unique examples in this book from children's hospitals worldwide, there will be many more exciting innovations.

Variable building components will give children greater control over their environments. Bedroom walls constructed of thin-screen video panels will envelop children in their favorite places—whether it is home, the ballpark, or on the family sailboat. Touch-screens and voice-activated controls will let children adjust the light, temperature, and acoustics of their spaces. Disney-like animatronics will be used in healing places, with interactive cartoon figures answering questions and giving directions in the elevator lobby.

Interactive networking and video will bring families, teachers, and healthcare providers together into a child's bedroom at home or in the hospital. Internet technology will keep parents with their children in the hospital, enabling them to work at the office or manage their home from their child's bedside. Holograms and voice recognition may allow physicians to work with multiple patients simultaneously in different locations, spreading their expertise and presence beyond the hospital. Wellness will be taught on information networks integrated into homes, schools, and healthcare environments. Hospital televisions will become information centers and educators, providing families and children with full access to healthcare, research, and wellness data.

Change will continue to be a constant as medicine, technology, finance, and new operational models evolve. Hospitals will care for more acutely ill children, while 23-hour facilities, outpatient centers, community clinics, and home care will provide the remainder of care. Modular interiors will facilitate daily changes in departmental layouts to respond to changing needs and support the efficient and continuous use of space. Information systems will provide data to measure the true outcomes of healthcare environments, providing feedback for future designs. Virtual reality simulators will walk design professionals, caregivers, family members, and children through healthcare environments before they are even built.

The unique identities of children's facilities will grow stronger on campuses as healthcare systems blur their cultures through corporate growth and acquisition. The patient-friendly achievements in children's care will eventually influence all healthcare facilities, bringing optimistic, interactive, and family-friendly environments to all ages.

**William Mead, AIA**
Shepley Bulfinch Richardson and Abbott
Boston MA

# USA State Abbreviations

| | | | | |
|---|---|---|---|---|
| Alabama | AL | | Montana | MT |
| Alaska | AK | | Nebraska | NE |
| Arizona | AZ | | Nevada | NV |
| Arkansas | AR | | New Hampshire | NH |
| California | CA | | New Jersey | NJ |
| Colorado | CO | | New Mexico | NM |
| Connecticut | CT | | New York | NY |
| Delaware | DE | | North Carolina | NC |
| District of Columbia | D.C. | | North Dakota | ND |
| Florida | FL | | Ohio | OH |
| Georgia | GA | | Oklahoma | OK |
| Hawaii | HI | | Oregon | OR |
| Idaho | ID | | Pennsylvania | PA |
| Illinois | IL | | Rhode Island | RI |
| Indiana | IN | | South Carolina | SC |
| Iowa | IA | | South Dakota | SD |
| Kansas | KS | | Tennessee | TN |
| Kentucky | KY | | Texas | TX |
| Louisiana | LA | | Utah | UT |
| Maryland | MD | | Vermont | VT |
| Massachusetts | MA | | Virginia | VA |
| Michigan | MI | | Washington | WA |
| Minnesota | MN | | West Virginia | WV |
| Mississippi | MS | | Wisconsin | WI |
| Missouri | MO | | Wyoming | WY |

# Acknowledgments

### Special Thanks

**Sara Marberry** - Sara Marberry Communications

**Lawrence A. McAndrews,** FACHE - National Association of Children's Hospitals and Related Institutions

**Laura Feldman** - National Association of Children's Hospitals and Related Institutions

**John and Brenda Fareri** - Children's Hospital Foundation, Westchester Medical Center

**Ronald W. Dennis,** AIA - HKS

**Joseph G. Sprague,** FAIA - HKS

**John I. Plappert,** AIA - Karlsberger Companies

**Linda M. Gabel,** IIDA - Karlsberger Companies

**Mitchel R. Levitt,** FMP - Karlsberger Companies

**John Pangrazio,** FAIA - NBBJ

**Rosalyn Cama,** FASID, ASID - President American Society of Interior Design

**Don Brunnquell** - Association for the Care of Children's Health

**Graham Nix** - United Bristol Healthcare NHS Trust

**David Hughes,** M.D. - United Bristol Healthcare NHS Trust

**William Mead,** AIA - Shepley Bulfinch Richardson and Abbott

**Gregory C. Mare,** AIA - NBBJ

**Bruce Bonine,** AIA - NBBJ

**Katie Komiske,** Newport RI

**Charleen Pysz** - Hasbro Children's Hospital, Providence RI

To all of the hospitals, designers, and photographers throughout the world that took the time and effort to share their accomplishments.

A very special thanks to HKS, Karlsberger Companies, NBBJ, and Shepley Bulfinch Richardson and Abbott for their support in the development of this book. They are all nationally recognized architectural firms who design contemporary pediatric healthcare environments.